Why Did I Just Eat That?

ENDORSEMENTS

"Lisa D. Ellis is masterful at conveying the necessary information to make fundamental, long-term, and meaningful change toward transforming our relationship with food. Her case studies, exercises, worksheets and activities are both user-friendly, informative, and facilitate true healing. Every part in *Why Did I Just Eat That?* includes incredible tips, strategies, and insights to change behavior and habits. She helps to create a path for her readers toward self-love, self-compassion, personal empowerment, and honoring who we are. I am elated for *Why Did I Just Eat That?* to be out there. Lisa truly hit the mark and so many people will undoubtably benefit."

Michelle Maidenberg, Ph.D., MPH, LCSW-R, CGP
Author of *Free Your Child from Overeating: A Handbook for Helping Kids and Teens* and *ACE Your Life: Unleash Your Best Self and Live the Life You Want*

"Lisa D. Ellis's *Why Did I Just Eat That?* is a beacon of understanding and support for those seeking to heal their relationship with food. With non-judgmental wisdom, she creates a safe space for readers to explore their eating issues and discover a path toward self-compassion, empowerment, and positive change."

Stacy Salob, MD

"Easy to read and relatable, *Why Did I Just Eat That?* gives practical tools for people to start their healing journey."

Lynn Green, MD

"*Why Did I Just Eat That?* is a motivating, heart-warming, and educational book full of inspiring information! For those who want to understand and make meaningful, values-driven steps towards a respectful relationship with their body and food, I highly recommend *Why Did I Just Eat That?*. Lisa D. Ellis does a phenomenal job creating a compassionate guide to change, which includes ways to be accountable and bolster self-reflection.

As Lisa integrates a systemic approach—family dynamics, physiology, psychology, and nutrition—the content is thoughtful, relatable, and well -organized. Using various interactive tools, such as metaphors, case studies, affirmations, and thought records, Lisa gently encourages readers to identify food messages/associations, alternative beliefs, essential emotions, and evolve perspectives. I appreciated how the information was validating and normalizing. I found this to be a refreshing and thoughtfully planned self-help book, and I was grateful for the humor and the consistent reminders to practice self-kindness!"

Laura Vraney, Psy.D.

WHY
Did I Just
Eat That?

How to Let Go of Emotional Eating
and Heal Your Relationship with Food

LISA D. ELLIS
MS, RDN, CDN, LCSW, CEDS-C

NEW YORK

LONDON • NASHVILLE • MELBOURNE • VANCOUVER

WHY Did I Just Eat That?

How to Let Go of Emotional Eating and Heal Your Relationship with Food

© 2024 Lisa D. Ellis, MS, RDN, CDN, LCSW, CEDS-C

The case studies presented in this book are intended to illustrate the principles and practices discussed. The names, identifying details, and specifics of the individuals mentioned have been changed to protect their privacy and confidentiality. The examples mentioned are composites of several individuals. Any resemblance to actual persons, living or dead, is purely coincidental.

This book is intended to provide information and guidance on nutrition, diet, eating intuitively, and healing one's relationship with food. The information contained in this book is not intended to replace medical advice, treatment, or diagnosis from a licensed healthcare professional. The advice provided in this book is based on the author's personal experience and research, and may not be suitable for everyone. Readers are advised to consult with a qualified healthcare provider before making any changes to their diet or lifestyle based on the information provided in this book, and otherwise use their own judgment and discretion when implementing any lifestyle or dietary changes.

Published in New York, New York, by Morgan James Publishing. Morgan James is a trademark of Morgan James, LLC. www.MorganJamesPublishing.com

Proudly distributed by Publishers Group West®

Morgan James BOGO™

A **FREE** ebook edition is available for you or a friend with the purchase of this print book.

_____

CLEARLY SIGN YOUR NAME ABOVE

Instructions to claim your free ebook edition:
1. Visit MorganJamesBOGO.com
2. Sign your name CLEARLY in the space above
3. Complete the form and submit a photo of this entire page
4. You or your friend can download the ebook to your preferred device

ISBN 9781636982090 paperback
ISBN 9781636982106 ebook
Library of Congress Control Number: 2023937234

Cover and Interior Design by:
Chris Treccani
www.3dogcreative.net

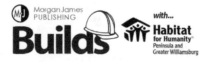

Morgan James is a proud partner of Habitat for Humanity Peninsula and Greater Williamsburg. Partners in building since 2006.

Get involved today! Visit: www.morgan-james-publishing.com/giving-back

*This book is dedicated to my husband and children
for supporting my career every step of the way.*

To CW, my partner in crime.

*To my mother, for teaching me early on in life the value of nourishing my body,
and my dad who modeled how to practice healthcare with compassion.*

*And, to my brother Jef, whose research in the connection between
anxiety and creativity helped inform part of the first section of this book,
and who supported me in making my dream a reality.*

TABLE OF CONTENTS

ACKNOWLEDGMENTS

Thanks to my interns—past and current—Rachel Dillon, Suzanne Appel Duffy, and Alexa Singman, for their creativity and assistance.

Thanks also to Beverley Delay who skillfully turned a manuscript into the first version of the real, live book, and to Elissa Held and Molly Kestenbaum for their creativity and artistic talents.

I am grateful to Nina Mattikow for her invaluable guidance and support.

I am likewise indebted to Bess Frankel, Rachel Glanz, Deborah Klein and Nadine Goldenberg Monaco, for their insight and suggestions.

And finally, this book is only possible because of the many clients I've had the privilege to counsel. I am so grateful they have trusted me in their food freedom journeys.

PREFACE

"Look at her! *This* is why we're here," the mother screamed as she grabbed hold of the belly of her pre-teen daughter, shaking it vigorously. "She hides food...and I can't watch her 24 hours a day!" The girl was barely 12 years old, sitting on my office couch, and sobbing next to her furious mother. Tears were falling onto the knees of her jeans in big, wet drops.

As a Registered Dietitian, I had never felt so powerless. What was I supposed to do, tell this despondent child to eat more celery and less cake, and then say, "Good luck, see you next week, when I'll give you more diet advice you'll do your best to ignore?" It was pretty clear her eating issues had less to do with nutrition than with the emotional and psychological issues she was struggling with. I felt woefully over-matched.

Also, I understood some of what the girl was experiencing.

I can remember my summer camp counselor giving seven-year-old me clear popsicles while the other kids were enjoying ice cream cones because, as she said, "Girls like us need to watch our figures."

Today, impressionable kids base their wrong-headed sense of self-worth on unrealistic posts found on Instagram and TikTok. For girls coming of age in the 1980s, however, we learned how we were *supposed* to look from teen magazines. So, it was through teen magazines that I first bought into what is now known as "diet culture." I learned all about minimizing calories and what foods I needed to avoid to look good in a bikini. My desperation to adhere to these standards overshadowed everything else in my life. My high school years were a joyless blur of comparisons, perfectionism, and disappointments, restricting and binging, fad diets, weight lost, and weight regained.

The struggles I endured had a lot to do with my choosing my profession. Health concerns aside, issues of weight and body shape in a society filled with negative judgment and unattainable beauty standards can often feel overwhelming, especially for women. I went to school to become a Registered Dietitian, hoping that as I learned to help others fix their bodies, I might learn to help myself. After all (I misguidedly believed at the time), the best way to love your body was to change it into something everyone else would envy. But, as I began my practice as an RD, it became frustratingly clear that diets rarely work long term. I could get my clients to take weight off but not to keep it off.

There was something profoundly moving about what the sobbing girl in my office was going through—she, and the many others like her, whose food intake issues are not addressed by nutrition science alone. And I had a flash of realization.

My first epiphany was that I needed to completely reject what we now refer to as "diet culture." There is no room for judgment, shaming, or coercion in the healing process. I began to investigate the causes of eating disorders and other unhealthy patterns of eating. I researched as much as I could: I reviewed dietitian trade journals as well as academic papers and studies by nutritionists and psychologists, more nuanced papers by neuroscientists and anthropologists, and many of the studies those papers cited. I consulted with psychologists and therapists and life coaches and then earned my own MSW (Master of Social Work) from Fordham University. It became very clear that the dynamics of food and eating (and our relationship to both) are as complex as any other major aspect of our lives, up there with personal relationships, sex, and money.

Eating disorders and eating issues, ranging from minor to potentially life-threatening, are symptoms of other, often much deeper, concerns. The purpose of this book is to identify the common, underlying causes of eating issues and give clarity to people struggling from them. When eating issues are demystified, they lose much of their influence. As the influence of these issues diminishes, the tools we discuss in this book can help empower you to begin to heal—and regain joy with—your relationship with food.

And with healing comes freedom — freedom from outdated assumptions, freedom from harmful self-talk. All you need is to find the way. Resolving these eating and food issues is a process. It takes observation and awareness and courage.

Let's do it together.

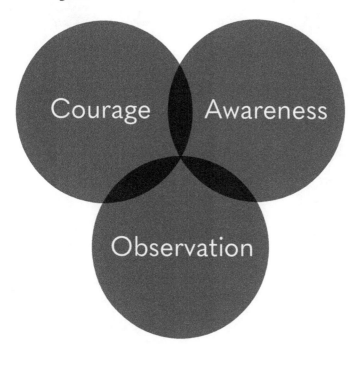

HOW TO GET THE MOST OUT OF THIS BOOK

W*hy Did I Just Eat That?* is divided into four parts, with downloadable workbook pages and other resources available online at https://whydidijusteatthat.com. The book starts with general information, followed by fictionalized case studies (each case is a composite of several different clients with all personal information changed to preserve privacy). The final part provides exercises and activities, including affirmation work, journaling, and brief workbook assignments.

I wholeheartedly suggest that people working on healing their relationship with food follow the path set out in this book. Read all of the background information and do the activities relevant to you to the best of your ability, remembering to always be gentle with yourself.

The **FIRST PART** of this book helps the reader gain insight on how our biology sets up *every human being* to have eating issues. Understanding the pre-programmed instincts we all share is an important part of learning how each of us can grow beyond habits that do not serve us. For many people, understanding the mechanics of a problem—the *why* of things—is an important part of mastering the issue and finding a path toward healing.

The **SECOND PART** is interactive and includes a brief quiz designed to help readers gain more specific insight into their own individual issues. It should take between 10 and 15 minutes to complete. This quiz narrows down the specific type(s) of eater the reader is, setting up the curative steps specific to each respective eater found in the third section.

The **THIRD PART** discusses strategies and suggested solutions for healing and growth, honoring and working with —and not against —the biological influences we're all born with, as well as the specific, idiosyncratic tendencies that affect the way each of us eats individually. The exercises and worksheets used here are the same that I've developed and successfully used in my practice.

And finally, **PART FOUR** discusses takeaways, helpful tips, and next steps after the reader has completed the first three sections.

Do make use of the book's dedicated website, https://whydidijusteatthat.com. Click on the RESOURCES tab, where you will find downloadable worksheets and a printable version of the Awareness Quiz, as well as additional tools and instructional videos; all designed to help you put into practice the lessons you will learn in this book.

INTRODUCTION

T he writer Leo Tolstoy famously wrote, "All happy families are alike; each unhappy family is unhappy in its own way," and this rings true, I think, about the relationship individuals have with food.

A person with a healthy, empowered relationship with food finds that food is something to be enjoyed, celebrated, or maybe is simply part of what one does each day. Food does not occupy a major place in their thoughts, and it certainly is not something they obsess and struggle over.

On the other hand, there are as many reasons for disempowered eating as there are disempowered eaters. Most of my nutrition counseling practice is working with disempowered eaters, and I have broken them down into categories with shared tendencies later in this book. But the one element many seem to have in common is that they feel powerless in the face of their struggle with Emotion-Triggered Eating. Much of this book is dedicated to dealing with the causes of Emotion-Triggered Eating, and more importantly, outlining ways to heal and move on from it.

What Is Emotion-Triggered Eating?

"The phrase "Emotional Eating" usually carries a negative meaning in our society. It suggests poor eating habits, unhealthy ways to cope with stress, and feelings of shame. (That description is the reason the term Emotional Eating is included in the subtitle of this book.) Yet this definition is a bit simplistic and not completely accurate. After all, enthusiastically enjoying a slice of cake to celebrate a joyful event might be described as emotional eating but is not necessarily a problem. On the other hand, if every time your mother calls, you find yourself automatically rooting through your cookie jar and eating multiple cookies without actually tasting them, that call could be accurately described as an Emotion Trigger and probably points to a problem. Which is why I believe that Emotion-Triggered Eating is a more accurate term when it comes to discussing certain eating issues. It points out that the emotion-trigger aspect is just as important as the eating aspect.

While some people's food choices are affected by how certain foods affect their bodies, many more struggle with emotional, psychological, and even spiritual issues that influence their eating habits. This is where the concept of Emotion-Triggered Eating comes in. Problematic Emotion-Triggered Eating behavior shows up in two contradictory forms: eating too much or eating too little. Eating too much in a specific period of time is binge eating; eating too little is known as food restriction. Each has its own payoff; each is an attempt to manage anxieties.

Binge eating can give the binge eater a sense of comfort, a sense of fullness amidst feelings of emptiness. (Some binge-eaters have described this feeling of being stuffed as feeling like they're "being hugged from within.") Food can perform like an old, dependable friend: comfortable, soothing, predictable.

At the other end of the spectrum, people who deliberately restrict can get a sense of manufactured well-being and false empowerment, a sense of control that reminds them, "I'm bigger than my hunger" with the peal of each hunger pang. The danger here is that the high walls of food restriction may eventually collapse into the rubble of anorexia.

When anorexia takes charge, people struggling with the condition restrict so much food that they actually lose contact with their own body's hunger cues, no longer following the natural instinct to eat. A related group of problematic eaters are bulimics, who take drastic measures to avoid weight gain, including vomiting and/or fasting after binge-eating, misusing laxatives and/or diuretics, and/or engaging in excessive exercise.

The Struggle of the Emotion-Triggered Eater

Whether binge eaters or restrictive eaters, people suffering from emotion-triggered eating often feel overwhelmed by their behavior. They often wallow in resulting feelings of shame and guilt, wanting badly to get past their disordered eating patterns but feeling trapped and unable to do so. Many also have an "all-or-nothing" attitude about their problem: *Eat perfectly, or why bother?* In that paradigm, the "nothing" of the all-or-nothing struggle wins; we beat ourselves up over food, give up, and surrender, only to end up with the exact opposite result from the one we had planned on. Namely, we end up with extra weight, less than an ideal weight, or compromised health.

So, with that in mind, the first thing to do is diminish the overwhelm by explaining why and how emotion-triggered eating occurs.

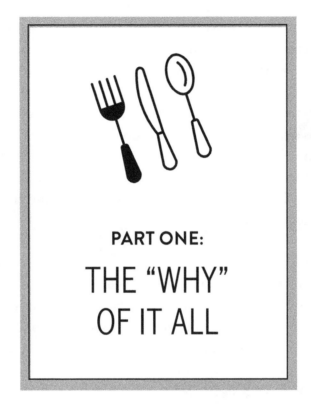

PART ONE:

THE "WHY"
OF IT ALL

As a culture, it is no exaggeration to say we're obsessed with two clashing interests: food on the one hand, and body shape and size on the other. The collision of foodie culture and weight obsession is brightly and loudly played out across the landscapes that surround us: TV, magazines, billboards, the vast social and digital media landscape, and our own homes. Food vs. weight; weight vs. food...no wonder we're overwhelmed!

That disconnect is part of the reason why it's likely you or somebody you know is struggling with their eating or body shape.

For some, this is a major problem.

In order to start healing these eating issues, we will first take a close look at them. The best way to solve any big problem, after all, is to break it down into understandable pieces.

We're Only Human

Like all biological creatures, we are vulnerable to our environment, and so to survive we use our senses to interact with our surroundings. We use our sense of sight to do things like guide us to safe paths, find food, and pick suitable people for mating purposes. Our ability to detect scents helps us avoid potentially dangerous things like smoke from a fire. Our hearing alerts us to potential dangers, like sounds of falling trees or the growl of a hungry tiger.

Our senses of taste and appetite help us discern what's good to eat from what isn't. In the most obvious cases, many things that are poisonous to us taste bitter, as our tastes developed to avoid such things. Rotting things contain dangerous bacteria and taste putrid to us so we are repulsed by them.

On the other hand, certain elements tend to be appealing to us. Fats, for example. Humans need a certain amount of fat to thrive. The average adult requires about 25 to 30 percent of daily caloric intake. (Pregnant and nursing mothers need a bit more fat, and babies and young children need more fat for their brains and neurological systems to develop properly.) Another appealing element is sugar. Sugar—in its natural, unrefined state, such as in fruit and honey—is helpful as an immediate energy source for the body.

In the earliest days of human existence, access to sugars and fats was limited. The wild animals available to our ancient ancestors were scrawnier than the domesticated animals we are familiar with today. Most wild fruits, before the age of agriculture, were likewise not as large or sweet as today's juicy fruits. Early hunter-gatherers lived in groups to maximize food-gathering potential, eating what they could find or catch. They lived in an environment of often unrelenting scarcity. They probably went hungry.

A lot.

To encourage a diet ensuring our species' continuity, certain brain chemicals guided us toward important food elements. *Dopamine* is activated in moments of pleasant surprise—such as the unexpected discovery of available food—and works in association with other brain chemicals known as *opioids*, which release feelings of pleasure. Since nutritious food was often scarce, finding sustenance with a lot of storable energy (like fats) and high in easily usable energy (calories) was critical; brain chemistry thus evolved to appreciate fats and sugars, two elements necessary for nutritional survival. Primal humans developed a taste for sugar and fats to encourage them to gather these comparatively rare nutrients. This drive to eat nutritious foods kept those early humans alive, making it possible for us—their modern descendants—to be here today.

But that same drive left us with a challenging legacy: we inherited an enduring taste for fatty, sweet things. That explains much of the inherent appeal we have for candy bars. When you consider that salt was another rare item for hunter gatherers (it is necessary in small amounts for things like transmitting nerve impulses, maintaining a proper fluid balance in the body, and optimum muscle operation), you begin to see why we are also hardwired to want potato chips!

Moreover, in the wild, carbohydrates and fiber are generally found together, with grains, beans, fruits and vegetables containing blends of both. In pre-modern times, if one wanted carbs, one would also get the important nutritional benefit of fiber, necessary for good health. But modern food processing often separates the two, creating an imbalance between carbs and fiber in the food choices of many people.

The evolutionary opioid-dopamine programming to seek out fatty, carby, sugary, and salty substances persists today, even though they are now widely available. We call this programming "craving."

Craving Ravings

So-called *junk food*—and food that isn't necessarily considered junk food, like bread and pasta—are foods that contain abundant elements our primal selves still crave. The downside is that these foods supply fats or simple carbs or sugars in larger portions than our ancient ancestors would find in the wild, often processed so that other nutritional elements—such as fiber—are removed.

These foods are designed to target our inherent cravings, but, of course, our bodies weren't designed to digest these elements in such excess. So while these foods feel satisfying, our diets can become unbalanced. Our cravings for food-based sugars, whole carbs, trace amounts of salt, and limited fats are satisfied by fast-food French fries that supply lots of these once-scarce nutrients in one massive, low-fiber serving. We wind up consuming more of these elements than we were ever designed to. The end result is the potential for seriously compromised health.

Yet cravings alone do not explain how Emotion-Triggered Eating works. That part of the puzzle, oddly enough, is linked to another set of primal self-survival mechanisms, most commonly known as "anxiety."

We tend to think of anxiety as an ongoing feeling of unease you just can't shake off (often unwarranted or exaggerated), connected to a vague impression that something is going to go wrong. Words associated with anxiety include "worry" and "nervousness." Ironically enough, a strong argument can be made that trying to quash feelings of anxiety can actually add to the anxiety already at work. The truth is, we all harbor some level of anxiety, because anxiety is a principle component of our survival mechanism system.

Anxiety as Defense Mechanism

If you have ever taken a walk through a park, you've likely noticed a squirrel or two making its way across the yard, dashing madly from tree to tree, running as fast as its little squirrel legs can carry it. A non-stop blend of cautious exploration and fearful reality checks. A frantic ballet of anxiety in action.

This "primal self/lizard brain" behavior has, of course, guaranteed the squirrel's survival. A squirrel that lazily saunters through the forest would make an easy snack for an owl and would probably get eaten before it could have genetically laid-back squirrel babies. A more hyper-aware, cautious squirrel would take care as it traveled, surviving long enough to have genetically hyper-aware, cautious babies. Through natural selection, eventually the descendants of all surviving squirrels are born to be vigilant and cautious.

The so-called "lizard brain" acts on basic urges and triggers reactions such as the fight-or-flight impulse that arises in moments of stress or danger. Honed over millions of years of evolutionary testing, the "lizard brain" is command central for the survival instinct.

The lizard brain aspect of our primal selves uses brain chemistry to achieve the goal of self-defense. In moments of perceived threat, a part of the brain called the hypothalamus sends a signal to the adrenal gland, which in turn relays a signal triggering the production of a steroid hormone called cortisol. Cortisol ramps up blood pressure and blood sugar levels; heart and breathing rates increase as the body prepares for a boost of energy for either battle or fleeing. Under the influence of cortisol, our awareness sharpens in order to focus on the perceived threat at hand, reducing our ability to regulate our emotions.

Since emotions and "feelings" are the main ways we interpret our experiences, when our emotions are under stress we are interpreting the relationship between ourselves and the world through an unreliable window. Because we can't successfully regulate our emotions during a stressful event, our emotions run haywire, often giving us an inaccurate picture of what's going on.

Moreover, when we are stressed by the trigger of some sort of threat, the part of the brain that exists for fight or flight takes charge (while the part responsible for higher thought is pushed out of the way). This explains why under stress we may feel scatterbrained. It's why you blanked and got questions wrong on tests at school when you actually knew the answers. It's also why stressed-out people can make poor, often self-sabotaging choices.

This dynamic is part of the reason people tend to stress-eat. But only part.

The Push-Pull of Emotion and Rationality

Emotions are felt and experienced. It is not their job to be rational. We have all had experiences where we reacted to something frustrating with an emotional outburst, even as our rational mind was thinking, *Well, that was the wrong way to respond to this situation.* (Road rage, anyone?) You might be wondering why our fight-or-flight response mechanism kicks in at simple confrontations that do not seem to be true threats.

The answer may surprise you: to that very primitive aspect of our mind system, every anxiety-related reaction comes from a deep-seated fear of death. Every phobia is rooted in a real—though often long-forgotten—life-or-death situation.

This includes things as innocent-seeming as social anxieties. Why should fear of—let's say—being embarrassed in front of peers be experienced as a life-or-death situation? Well, early humans depended on their tribes and families for cooperation in gathering food, establishing shelters, and for protection. For these ancient people, being shunned by the tribe could lead to banishment. Banishment from the tribe meant exile and exposure to the threats of the outside world: starvation, vulnerability to the outdoor elements, and danger from other tribes or predators. Though having a falling-out with our social groups no longer leads to mortal peril, we have a deep-seated need to feel socially accepted that has been inherited over countless generations. To the primal self, social ostracization equals abandonment and potential death...and that instinctual fear has echoes today. Even in high school. Especially in high school.

Likewise, a fight with your boss might trigger fears rooted in life-or-death vulnerability: annoy your boss, lose your job, lose your ability to survive.

When feeling at all at risk, the primal self uses our emotions to trigger what the lizard brain considers to be appropriate actions. Obviously, emotions urging us to either fight or flee are rarely appropriate responses to everyday challenges in our lives. When the energy that's made available for us to engage or to run isn't used, the bottled-up fight-or-flight energy has to go *somewhere*. This is often experienced as frustration. Or stress. Or feelings of enhanced anxiety. The longer these feelings swirl around, the more they build up inside of us.

We've all had an argument with someone over the phone. The call ends, but our emotional energy is in full gear, heart rate up in full fight or flight mode. But we continue to sit at our desk and try to focus on whatever task is at hand, as the emotional upset is churning around inside. It becomes a little more difficult to concentrate, and the irritation at that only adds to the overall emotional darkness. We get annoyed at ourselves for being annoyed. Maybe we yell at the dog, and regret it immediately.

Soon that feeling fades. But it doesn't completely go away.

And so a background level of ongoing anxiety from unresolved emotional responses becomes our typical way of being. We don't even notice it.

Because anxiety comes from a sense of survival insecurity, moments of elevated anxiety trigger a kind of survival mode. We are compelled to obtain things that make us feel secure—warm, safe, protected. We yearn to be soothed with assurances to the lizard brain that our survival is not actually at risk. We crave things that are consistent with our most elemental means of survival.

In other words, we want to be comforted.

This is where the need for comfort food is rooted.

Since human beings have the inherited programming to actively seek out fats, carbs, and sugars to feel fortified and ready for battle—and a whole range of even minor social and cultural conflicts between people can literally feel like life-and-death incidents to our inner, primal selves—it is no mystery why certain emotional responses to even routine conflicts trigger an impulse to reach for these food elements in many people.

Food is popular as a comfort mechanism because it actually can create the illusion of achieving both ends, numbing *and* control. Food is also an easy form of comfort because it's available everywhere.

We are all familiar with what can be soothing about comfort foods—the pleasures those foods offer that our primal selves instinctively crave: sweet tastes, salty tastes, and creamy mouthfeel. Consider the tummy-filling satisfaction of high-carb foods like bread and mashed potatoes, usually served with generous dollops of fats like butter or cream. Breads (carbs) are often served with butter (fats) or peanut butter (fats and, often, sugars) and jelly (sugars). Cake offers one-stop food satisfaction, providing loads of carbs and fats and sugars. "Yummy yum yum," says our primal self.

A feeling of a full belly, too, can have a comforting effect. In times of emotional insecurity, the full tummy sensation can elicit a feeling of completeness, a sort of money-in-the-bank feeling to counteract a sense of emotional lack. If we felt safe as children, we may associate sensations of feeling safe when we eat the same food we ate when we were small.

One noteworthy source of anxiety is past trauma, and many people dealing with trauma find comfort in food. It is not unusual to see victims of sexual abuse struggling with eating issues. There is also mounting evidence that previous trauma can actually be passed from parent to child epigenetically (that is, transferred to the next generations by a means other than altered DNA) and this dynamic can span multiple generations. What this means is that we can have a level of anxiety stemming from traumas that we, ourselves, never actually experienced, from events whose memories have long since been erased by time. As strange as it seems, a need for comfort may not be related to any concrete event in the life of the person seeking that comfort.

Finally, food can also appear to be empowering. When we buy food, or order a meal, or prepare a snack, we are exerting at least a little control over our lives. We are in charge of what we choose to eat, even if we know it is not in alignment with our nutrition goals.. The battle between some parents and children over how much or how little the kids eat is also a battle of control.

If we view all of this under a single umbrella, we might see achieving comfort—as it relates to food, among other things—as a strategy-based method one can take to deal with anxieties. Comfort can come from not only food, but other sources as well: hugs, a hot bath, a phone call from a good friend, a TV sitcom, even cushioned bedroom slippers. Comfort soothes our primal selves with a sense of control and protection.

And that's where the emotion-triggered eating problem starts.

The Primal Self and the Irrelevance of Reality

The primal self has no sense of context and is actually unaware of the passage of time. It is reactive, and operates on feelings and impressions. That is why an event that made us angry in the past can—given enough thought and energy—make us angry in the present. How many of us can reignite upset feelings by recalling elementary school conflicts...even decades later? Since these feelings can persist even if the inciting event is forgotten or misremembered, it becomes clear how anxieties sparked by events that took place years ago might still have a hold on us today. So, it is pretty likely we are carrying a level of anxiety that has no real connection to our current lives. Even more alarming, when our primal selves shift into fight-or-flight mode and we don't start fighting or fleeing, our anxiety level escalates. Add to that any real worries we might have, and wow! That's a lot of emotional baggage for anyone to bear.

The Takeaway

When the primal self feels vulnerable and at risk, it will do all it can to feel safe. That is its job. Unfortunately, it cannot distinguish between the anxiety of having no food and the common emotional anxiety that something is missing from one's life. It also equates any sort of social conflict with a potentially life-threatening tribal isolation. Moments of even minor distress ramp up anxiety, and as anxiety ramps up, so do levels of cortisol. When cortisol levels elevate, the primal self craves calorie-dense foods in order to be ready to fight for its life or literally run for cover. And after the perceived threat has passed, cortisol acts to replenish energy supplies spent during the fight-or-flight response, no matter how little energy was actually expended.

What that means is that in moments of stress, we crave carbohydrates, sugar, and fatty foods, and in the moments following stress, we crave carbohydrates, sugar, and fatty foods. These food cravings feel uncomfortable, which is why satisfying the food cravings the cortisol demands actually has a soothing effect on us. Eating the desired foods triggers chemical changes that halt the cravings. Moreover, to deny these physical cravings may actually exacerbate the anxiety.

This is the root of stress eating.

Add to that the psychological dynamics of using food for comfort, and suddenly the concept of emotion-triggered eating makes tons of sense.

Our relationship with food mirrors the relationship we have with ourselves. That's potentially good news because this mirror goes two ways. If we can meaningfully change our relationship with food, the relationship we have with ourselves will shift as well. Change our relationship with ourselves, and the role food plays in our lives shifts as well. It is—if you'll forgive the food-related metaphor—a chicken-and-egg situation.

Too many of us feel disconnected from our own bodies, while putting pressure upon ourselves to change these bodies. We tend to be unaware of the major role genetic programming plays in what we want to eat, or the role of anxiety in overeating. Too many of us succumb to self-imposed pressure to change, pressure that leads to (no surprise) added anxiety, anxiety that compounds and ends in self-shaming, guilt, and self-loathing. Too many of us don't recognize that these issues are not rooted in our character flaws or insecurities, but our actual biology!

So, if you are suffering from any sort of eating issue, you might find some solace in acknowledging that it is not your fault.

It is up to you, however, to transcend it.

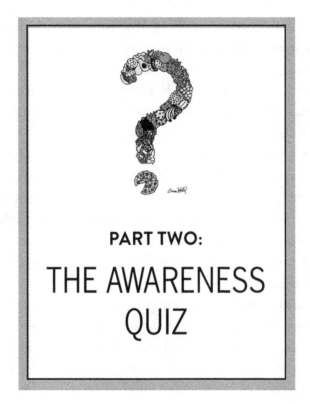

PART TWO:

THE AWARENESS QUIZ

wrote this book to help you, dear reader, help yourself heal your relationship with food. The purpose of Part 1 (the previous section) was to give you general information about eating issue dynamics that we all have in common; It puts everything in a wider context. The purpose of Part 2 (this section) is to help you zoom on specific information about your own eating issue dynamics.

To get the most from this book, I recommend you take the following quiz, and then follow up by participating in the appropriate workbook exercises as indicated. (More on that a little later.)

There is a saying in therapeutic and personal growth circles that I often reflect upon while working with my clients: "Simple awareness is often curative." While I don't believe the people I see would be immediately healed of all of their eating and body image issues solely through awareness of their particular habits and triggers, awareness is an important first step toward breaking through the blocks that have many feeling trapped and hopeless.

There are as many types of eating issues as there are types of people. Over the years, I have noticed that there are certain tendencies that show up in individuals as specific eater types—different personalities grouped around kinds of behavior related to eating and food. The good news is that there are ways to directly and specifically address these individual eating issues.The purpose of this quiz, then, is to help you identify the type of eater you are.

As you take the quiz, bear in mind that while most of the concepts listed may feel a little true for you some of the time, other statements will jump out as being major tendencies most or all of the time, and these are the statements you might pay close attention to. Of course, there are no right or wrong choices, and the purpose of this is to help you guide yourself toward greater self-awareness as a tool to use in your healing process.

Before starting the quiz, it is important to remember that it is natural for emotions to affect our eating. It's absolutely fine, from time to time, to indulge in the pure joy of savoring food, even if it means going beyond mere fullness. By the same token, a joyful wedding toast or celebrating the birthday of a loved one by having a slice of cake can easily fall into the category of consuming food with great emotion. So is eating a plate of food that was your favorite as a child because you are feeling nostalgic or homesick. For someone going through a painful breakup, eating hot fudge sundaes as part of their emotional recovery is a perfectly normal and common way of seeking solace. These behaviors are worrisome only when they become the primary way of expressing or dealing with emotions, and when such behavior becomes chronic and threatens good health or mindful, daily functioning.

What Type of Eater Are You?

To get the most out of this quiz, read the statements below, and select those that apply to you by putting a check in the blank space at the beginning of the sentence. (While many of these statements may be true some of the time, take care to focus on those that are typically true of you more often than not.) When you are finished, there will be further instructions on how to score your responses by counting and then tallying the individual symbol shapes next to the statements you selected. Please allow around 15 minutes to take this test.

For a printable version of this quiz, visit www.whydidijusteatthat.com/resources for your downloadable copy.

1. I struggle with making self-care a priority for myself. It is much easier for me to take care of people other than myself. ■ ▲
2. I regularly use food for comfort; it makes me feel better. ♥ ☽
3. If I eat "bad" foods, I am doing a bad thing, or consider myself a bad person. ▲
4. When I eat (or restrict myself from eating) food, and that goes against the wishes of other people, I feel more powerful. ■
5. I find myself nibbling on food all day, sometimes not making time for actual, proper, meals. ★ ☽ ●
6. There are times when I eat food—even though I may not feel hungry—that I feel obligated to eat anyway. ★

7. I often use eating to get back at others by consuming foods I think I should not eat. ■

8. I feel guilty and bad about myself if I do not exercise regularly. ▲

9. When I feel angry at someone and don't feel comfortable confronting them, I really want to eat. ♥ ■

10. I use food as a way to soothe my feelings when I'm feeling sad. ♥ ☽

11. I have feelings of disgust or loathing when I look at my body in the mirror. ▲

12. I eat throughout the day, and therefore rarely feel hungry. ★ ●

13. I often use food as a way to procrastinate getting tasks done. ☽

14. Sometimes I eat just because I know someone would disapprove of the fact that I was eating. ■

15. I eat as much as I can at a sitting because I'm afraid there won't be enough food later. ★

16. When it comes to sweets, I either eat the entire container or I eat none. ▲

17. I'd call myself a "grazer"; I snack frequently instead of eating meals. ☽ ●

18. I work out solely to change my body size and shape. ▲

19. Eating has a calming effect on me. ♥

20. I rarely plan out any meals or snacks in advance. ●

21. Eating helps me feel in control. ■

22. I impulsively grab food without considering if I'm hungry or not. ★ ☽

23. Normal stomach distention after eating makes me hate the way my body looks. ▲

24. My meals and snacks are at irregular times each day; sometimes I even skip them. ●

25. When I feel overwhelmed I find myself looking for food as comfort. ♥ ☽

26. I eat little during the day, but then eat continuously from dinner until bedtime. ●

27. I get most of my joy in life from eating. ♥ ★ ■
28. I frequently find myself eating when cleaning the kitchen. ♥ ★ ▲
29. I'm most often not hungry for breakfast or lunch and rarely eat much before dinner. ●
30. As a child, I would be offered a treat/sweet to help me feel better whenever I was upset. ♥ ☽
31. I have my list of "good" foods and "bad" foods that I follow. ▲
32. It matters little if I am full or not if the food looks good. ★
33. Growing up, I was expected to be part of the "clean plate club" (grown-ups did not allow me to leave any food on my plate.) ★ ▲
34. I know my loved one wants me to lose weight, so I eat to get back at them. ■
35. I might be full, but if there's food on my plate I will finish it! ★ ▲
36. I tend to eat a large dinner after eating very little throughout the day. ●
37. During more difficult days, I look for food to relieve the stress. ♥ ☽
38. I have no idea what I will eat until I open the fridge. ★ ●
39. I make food choices based on how good I feel about my body at that moment. ▲
40. I am a fast eater. ♥ ★ ■
41. I drink coffee all day and only eat food at night. ●
42. Eating is a great way for me to put off doing something I don't want to do. ♥ ■ ☽
43. When I feel stressed or upset I turn to food for relief. ■ ☽
44. I use the diet rules or internet "hacks" I find on social media as a guide to tell me what I should and should not eat. ▲
45. I believe it's my job to keep my family calm and happy. ■ ●
46. When I feel stressed I start looking for things to eat even if I'm not hungry. ♥ ☽
47. If I eat "bad" foods, I will not like the way my body looks. ▲
48. I notice that when I don't sleep well I look for more food. ●

49. I use food as a way to express resentment if I'm upset with certain people. ■

50. I try to be really "good" by not eating breakfast or lunch, even though I might be hungry. ▲ ●

51. I am compelled to eat everything on my plate regardless of how hungry (or not) I might feel. ★

52. I find I'm often way too busy during the workday for proper meals. ☽ ●

53. My problems would go away only if I could lose weight. In fact, my life would be perfect if I were in a smaller body. ▲

54. Eating comfort foods makes me feel better. ♥

55. I let myself have dessert only if I work out a lot that day. ▲

56. I ignore my feelings of hunger even though I'm aware that I feel hungry. ▲ ●

57. I usually try to be the first one at the table/in line for food. ♥ ★

58. I find I often anger-eat. ■

59. If I eat one cookie, I feel like my "diet" is ruined. ▲

60. When I feel tired, I grab food for energy and to make me feel more alert. ●

61. I will finish whatever uneaten food my kids leave on their plates, regardless of whether I'm hungry or not. ♥ ★ ●

62. I tend to eat if food is in front of me even if I'm not hungry. ★ ☽

63. I hide forbidden foods in secret places. ♥ ■

64. I either eat completely healthy, or just give up trying to eat healthy altogether. ▲

65. I believe it is better to finish food you don't want than to let it go to waste. ♥ ★ ●

66. I use over-eating as my way of expressing the uncomfortable feelings I have a hard time expressing. ■

67. When I have a poor night's sleep, I'm more likely to reach for extra snacks during the day. ●

68. When I feel lonely, food is my friend. ♥

69. I run out of energy in the middle of the day and use food as a pick-me-up. ●
70. The amount I exercise is based on working off what I eat. ▲
71. Other people don't understand how emotionally important food is to me. ❤
72. Not finishing everything on my plate makes me feel uneasy. ❤ ★
73. I'm always comparing my body to others. ▲
74. Being extra-full feels like I'm getting a hug from the inside. ❤ ■
75. Since food was scarce when I was younger, I carry concerns that there might not be enough to eat with me today. ★
76. I'm so busy taking care of my family that I put my own needs aside. ■ ●
77. I often tell myself "just one more snack and then I'll start my work." ☽
78. Food is a way for me to "numb out"/escape my real feelings. ❤ ☽
79. I carry anger and resentments I can't (or don't feel comfortable to) talk about. ■
80. I let what is put/served on my plate determine how much I will eat. ★
81. I have a hard time finishing assignments or chores because I get bored and eat instead. ☽
82. I grew up learning to sacrifice my needs for my family. ■ ●
83. Even after I'm full, if I see a food I like I will eat it. ★
84. If I eat something I consider "bad," I tell myself I'll start my diet on another day. ▲
85. If someone tells me not to eat something, it just makes me want it more. ■
86. When it comes to prioritizing all the things I have to do, I tend to put myself and my needs last on the list. ☽ ●

SCORING

When scoring, count the total number of symbols ({❤}, {■}, {▲}, {★}, {☽}, {●}) next to the statements with which you most identify. If there is more than one symbol next to a statement you select, make sure you tally all those symbols in your scoring. Then, in the **Eater Categories** section, read about each eater in the section or sections bearing the symbols you have selected most frequently.

Follow the action steps of the specific eater that most fits you and your concerns. If you find that statements describing more than one eater apply to you, I suggest you take the action steps of the Eater that is *most* present in your life, followed by any others in descending order of concern to you.

The purpose of this quiz is to help readers find the categories of eating issue tendencies that most closely corroborate with their relationship to food and eating. Please note that each of us is different, of course, and even people who share similar tendencies about their eating styles are unique individuals. No one—whether they struggle with severe eating issues, minor eating issues, or no eating issues at all—is purely one type of eater. We are all a blend of different and competing concerns and motivations.

EATER CATEGORIES

{1} Heart Group

The Food Cuddler

The options small children have in processing emotional challenges are pretty limited. Many find comfort in food, and as they grow into adulthood, this sense of being soothed by food stays with them. For Food Cuddlers, food serves as a main source of comfort, and occupies much of their awareness as they navigate their world.

The Pressure-Cooker Eater

Some people find they lose their appetites when upset, while others crave an overabundance of food. For too many people, stress is an ongoing problem that wreaks havoc on their relationship with food, whether they eat too little or try to soothe themselves by consuming way too much.

{2} Star Group

The Clean-Plate Eater

Clean Plate eaters feel obligated to eat everything on their plates—whether or not they are hungry—out of a well-meaning belief that we should never waste food. This feeling of obligation tends to create an out-of-balance relationship with food.

The Get-It-While-You-Can Eater

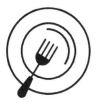

People who grew up with feelings of scarcity may find that feelings of never having enough to eat persist well after the causes of these feelings were an issue. For too many people, food satisfies the gut-level desire for abundance and security. While for many eaters, food is often a go-to source of comfort, The Get-It-While-You-Can Eater has a tendency to engage in emotionally triggered eating because of ongoing anxieties stemming from feelings of not having enough.

The See-Food Eater

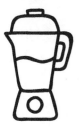

The See-Food Eater feels prompted to eat simply by being exposed to available, tempting foods. They often find the sight and smell, and even the sound of food sizzling, appetizing enough to impulsively want to eat that item—even if they are already full from a previous meal.

{3} Square Group

The Food Whisperer

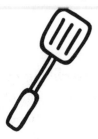 Some people are not able—or do not feel comfortable enough—to express themselves through direct communication. Food Whisperers find they signal displeasure through their eating habits, often stifling their emotions either through stress overeating or through drastically restricting their intake of food.

The Rebellious Eater

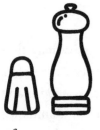 Much like the Food Whisperer, the Rebellious Eater uses food as a type of communication, consuming or restricting their intake of food as a way to say, "I control my body," when so much else seems beyond their control. What makes the habits of Rebellious Eaters more worrisome is that their food-use behavior can be more self-destructive,

often eating as a form of self-harm to express their unhappiness, anger, or dissatisfaction.

{4} Triangle Group

The All-or-Nothing-Eater

 All-or-nothing eaters frame eating habits in extremes, judging their eating choices in strictly opposing terms. Their philosophy: You either do your diet with complete, 100 percent perfection...or you just bail on it totally.

Food-Fad Eater

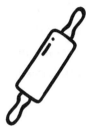

Many people follow strict, highly structured "fad" diets promoting sudden, drastic changes because they feel like something is out of control with their eating. But these diets are not sustainable in the long run, and going on and off fad diets (also known as yo-yo dieting) most often results in the opposite outcomes of what was intended.

{5} Crescent Group

The Procrastin-Eater

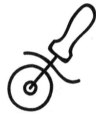

The Procrastin-Eater uses food as a distraction to avoid work or a pressing obligation. Some people use eating something as a way to put off starting a task or project they actually *want* to do, but don't know where or how to start. This becomes a more significant problem when they use food as the go-to coping mechanism whenever they are faced with a task. (Very often, this eating issue shows up in combination with another issue or two; I recommend each issue be addressed one at a time.)

{6} Circle Group

The Less-Mindful Eater

Less Mindful eaters tend to have no fixed meal or snack schedule, and few (if any) coherent eating strategies. They may be disconnected to the times when their hunger has been satisfied, often eating on a kind of autopilot, sometimes unconsciously consuming until they feel overstuffed.

The Less-Structured Eater

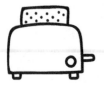

Some people feel that the lack of defined daily structure is freeing and so they use no food guideline strategies. But taken too far, a state of "no structure" sets up more challenges than setting reasonable boundaries...in nutrition, as well as in other aspects of day-to-day life.

Once-a-Day Diner

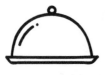

The Once-a-Day Diner will customarily eat little to no breakfast, little to no lunch—in fact, aside from maybe coffee and a trip to the vending machine, little or no food at all—until they get home from work famished and then pretty much eat everything in sight for the next few hours.

The Pendulum Eater

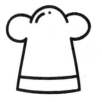

Some types of eaters are always looking for the next great diet, the next guaranteed way to shed pounds quickly, swinging from restrictive diet plan to restrictive diet plan, often losing weight, only to regain that weight and then some. Others see-saw back and-forth between harsh restriction and binge eating, then it's back to restrictive eating once again. What all Pendulum Eaters have in common is a wildly inconsistent relationship with food.

The Sleep-Deprived Snacker

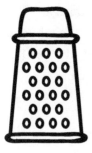

Many people use food as a way to compensate for inadequate sleep. During times when they don't get enough sleep, the Sleep-Deprived Snacker is liable to eat more food than usual to take in extra energy to help their lagging bodies stay awake. Moreover, tired people tend to eat more than is actually required due to their fatigue-impaired judgment.

The Taking-Care-of-Everyone-but-Me Eater

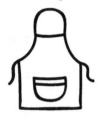

Too many people see simple self-care as somewhat frivolous, something to be pushed aside when there are so many other pressing issues to attend to. But not allowing ourselves time to meet our basic needs tends to leave us feeling depleted, and the Taking-Care-of-Everyone-but-Me Eater may regularly try to keep going by absentmindedly filling up with whatever food is quick and close at hand...and not necessarily the best choices.

NUTRITION BYTE: Whether restricting because of the latest fad diet, or restricting because of the newest health food currently in vogue, restricting what you allow yourself to eat keeps you from a wider range of nutrition choices and experiences.

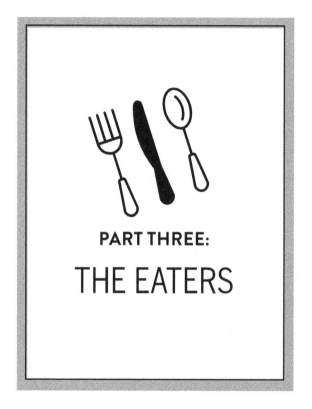

PART THREE:

THE EATERS

1

THE ALL-OR-NOTHING EATER

I t probably would not come as a great shock to anyone if I were to point out that there is often a connection between eating issues and some level of anxiety. I'm not just referring to major, clinical bouts of anxiety; I also refer to those garden-variety nagging sensations that can plague us all from time to time.

One of the ways we tend to manage our anxieties is by trying to control as many aspects of our lives as we can. The impulse to control often shows up in the form of perfectionism. And perfectionism is a major trigger of All-or-Nothing eating issues—because perfectionism and all-or-nothing eating both tend to have rigid, absolutist thinking at their roots.

The all-or-nothing mindset views eating choices in strictly opposing terms. You either do your diet with complete, 100 percent perfection, or you bail on it totally. One of my clients, a mom and middle-school schoolteacher named Sally (not her real name, of course) is a prime example of this dynamic.

THE ALL-OR-NOTHING EATER

Sally had been struggling with diets since she had her last child four years before she came to my office. At our first session, she mentioned an event that had happened the weekend before, which revealed her all-or-nothing approach to eating:

"I went out for Sunday brunch with my family, something I had been dreading all week. And they all wanted and ordered croissants. I wanted a croissant too, but I'm not allowed to have that on my diet, so I ordered an egg white omelet with tomato slices. I ate my food with my mouth, but theirs with my eyes. We went home and I felt so deprived that I began to eat a cookie...which turned into three, then eight, then the whole box. That's when the "f*ck-its" came in...I had already ruined my diet so I might as well eat everything I could find."

And so began a large binge. Sally ended her day feeling defeated once again.

This commitment to "be perfect or give up" is filled with good-intentioned but faulty thinking. Unless there is some sort of worrisome food allergy present, what is the harm of having, say, half a croissant with fruit—or even a whole one—if the alternative leads to an almost debilitating feeling of deprivation?

People who struggle with all-or-nothing eating see restriction as totally good, and the inevitable surrender to eating when you can't sustain perfection as totally horrible. As is the case with most people dealing with eating issues, the first step in healing a relationship with food is to stop being afraid of it.

One way to stop being afraid of this is to move our relationship with food from our rule-based mind to our intuitive heart. I'm a firm believer in Intuitive Eating, an important pillar of which is following your hunger and fullness cues. With Intuitive Eating, we don't see restricting food as a good thing in and of itself. And most importantly, an Intuitive Eater enjoys eating and respects food as a good thing...without guilt or misgivings.

And my final tip to taking the power out of all-or-nothing thinking—whether the subject is food, or any other aspect of our lives where crippling perfectionism rears its ugly head—is to remember that in most cases, good enough is good enough.

So why don't we give ourselves a break, embrace the "good enough," and trust our intuition? If we can do that, finding our way around Sunday brunch just may get a bit easier.

Self-Correction Toolkit for the All-or-Nothing Eater

> To gain the greatest benefit from this toolkit, I highly recommend you obtain a dedicated notebook to do your work in, or download our toolkit worksheets by visiting www.whydidijusteatthat.com/resources and click on the "All-or-Nothing Eater" link for printable copies.

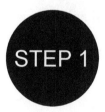

ADMIT...THEN COMMIT

All-or-nothing eating is rooted in all-or-nothing thinking. The good news is that with some work, virtually anyone can shift from inflexible, all-or-nothing thinking to a more flexible mindset.

Write a Starting-Point Affirmation

Admit that you understand, for your highest good, that there needs to be a change in your style of thinking. Take some quiet time to acknowledge this, then record your thoughts as an affirmation in your notebook or downloaded workbook pages You might write down, "I am moving toward a more flexible mindset," to record your affirmation, then sign and date it. I also recommend finding a moment to look in the mirror and tell yourself this intention, explaining why—in your own words—this is important to you.

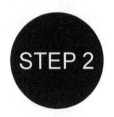

OBSERVE

Observe. That's all.

Just pay attention to your reactions throughout your day, especially the things that trigger emotionally charged thoughts or opinions. Are your reactions appropriate and your attitudes rational, or are they based on old habits of thinking that no longer serve you? The answers to this question are not as important as simply exercising your self-reflection skills.

Some Typical All-or-Nothing Thought Examples

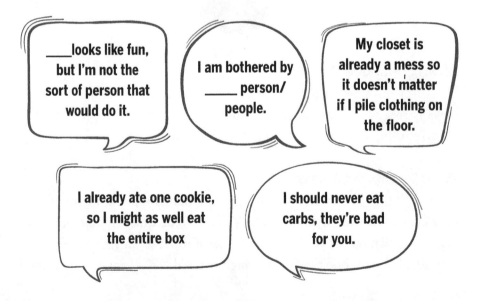

Observing Your All-or-Nothing Thoughts

Now it's your turn to put your focus on your own All-or-Nothing thoughts. Keep track of these thoughts in your notebook, downloaded workbook pages, or open a list application in your smartphone, tablet, or computer. (Pay specific attention to the all-or-nothing thoughts you have about food, but any all-or-nothing thinking is relevant.)

Take your time with this process and be gentle with yourself if you identify trends about your thinking that you realize you don't like. Spend a few days tracking your thoughts; don't judge, simply bring your attention to your thoughts. After you get a firm sense of whatever inflexible dynamics show up in your own thinking, go on to the next section.

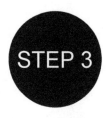

REWORK AND REFRAME

The goal of this exercise is to help you move from an all-or-nothing approach toward a more integrative way of thinking. Now that you have spent some time gathering your all-or-nothing thoughts for Step Two, it is time for you to rework and reframe your previous, limiting thinking.

Here are the examples I offered from Step Two, now reworked and reframed by adding new strategies:

Joining a book club looks like fun, but I'm not the sort of person who would do that.

Joining a book club looks like fun, though it has never occurred to me to join one. Maybe I should look into it. Merely checking something out does not obligate me to do anything, but it might open up opportunities for me that I was not aware of. I know I tell myself that I don't have the time, but is that totally true?

I already ate one cookie, so I might as well eat the entire box.

I ate one cookie, and I am glad I did because it was yummy. Perhaps, I'll have one or two more. Or, I might save them for another time when I want a tasty treat.

I am bothered by

_____

I am bothered by _____ person/people, but I realize that I don't really know them, or understand that thing about them that triggers such a reaction in me. Maybe I should give that some thought.

My closet is already a mess so it doesn't matter if I pile clothing on the floor.

Even though my closet is a mess, if I drop this clothing on the floor my space will become even messier. I'm going to have to hang it up or put it in the dirty laundry at some point anyway, so I'll start that now.

I should never eat carbs, they're bad for you

There is no such thing as bad food, unless it is moldy or spoiled or in some other way toxic. Bodies need some amount of carbs to be healthy. For my eating strategy, it is a good idea to not eat more carbs than what feels right in my body.

Now it's your turn! Copy your own All-or-Nothing thoughts into your notebook or workbook pages. To each one, add strategies that reflect a more flexible and less limiting way of thinking.

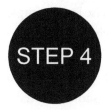

STEP 4

CHALLENGING THE CRITICAL VOICE

We've put some effort into identifying all-or-nothing thinking and exercising a more flexible approach to thinking by questioning some of our assumptions. Step Four takes the exploration of our assumptions to a deeper level, pushing back against the harsh assumptions we make against ourselves. These assumptions are also known as **self-judgments**.

As a side note, self-judgments are different from the sort of judgments that people make all the time, such as "I like that shirt," or, "I don't like that hairstyle." These are more preferences than judgments. Moreover, self-judgments—which carry negative energy—are different from self-assessments, which are emotionally neutral. You might, for instance, self-assess that you are good at one thing and not so good at another thing and yet not feel particularly positive or negative about these assessments. But if you dump negative thoughts all over yourself due to some perceived shortcoming, that is a judgment.

The word "should" feeds the negativity associated with harsh self-judgments. This dynamic exists when someone thinks, *I should drink six cups of water a day*, or, *I should exercise daily*, and if they don't do these things they judge themselves for messing up.

When we judge ourselves, or when we impose a "should" upon ourselves and then don't follow up on that "should," we often feel shame and/or guilt. Both shame and guilt are self-imposed negative mechanisms we use to punish ourselves. This is especially true for an inflexible, all-or-nothing thinker. They use the painful feelings of shame and guilt to beat themselves up; the payoff is that they can still feel like a good person even though they did something they consider to be bad, because they are punishing themselves for their bad behavior.

So for **Step Four**, the exercise is very simple. Observe how many times you catch yourself saying or thinking "I should," or making a negative judgment about yourself.

What were these "should" statements you have imposed upon yourself? Every time you say or think a "should" statement add a tally mark next to the statement.

Are there "should" statements that would be better for you to let go of? In your notebook or workbook, write down a commitment to yourself that you are letting go of those "shoulds." Be specific about what "shoulds" you are releasing.

Are there "should" statements you would like to keep, but need to renegotiate when or how or where you will work on them? In your notebook or workbook, write down the specific "should" you chose to renegotiate and what the renegotiations bring about.

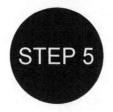

AFFIRM WHO YOU ARE

We opened these exercises with one affirmation, and we will close them with another. This final step is an ongoing process to take firm ownership of a more flexible way of interacting with your world.

In your notebook or workbook, write down the following statement, putting your name in the provided blank space:

I am _____. My heart is open, my attitude is flexible, and I gracefully forgive myself for being imperfect. I am enough, and worthy just as I am now.

Try to repeat your new affirmation to yourself every day in quiet moments, perhaps as you lie in bed in the morning or at the end of your day, or while meditating or exercising. Try to do this every day for at least a month. If you forget, that's fine, just forgive yourself and pick up where you left off. Even if you don't fully believe this statement at first, remember that in order to grow, we must become clear on what we aspire to be.

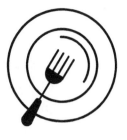

2

THE CLEAN-PLATE EATER

I t can be a challenge to dismiss the messages we got from our parents when we were young. Even the ones that no longer serve us can linger for years if we let them go unquestioned. The challenge with being this kind of eater is that the deep-rooted habit is often so ingrained in our way of eating that it becomes difficult to change.

THE CLEAN-PLATE EATER

Many of us were encouraged to join a very special club when we were small. This encouragement came from parents, grandparents, babysitters, teachers, and other caregivers. As far as I know, this special club wasn't all that exclusive; in fact there was only one criterion for membership: you had to completely clean your plate. It was, of course, "The Clean-Plate Club." The rules were pretty simple: *If it's in front of you, you gotta eat it!*

After all, your parents worked hard to buy you that food, and it was a sin to waste it. I can remember one time, around first grade, when the well-meaning parent of a friend told us kids that we had to finish our plates, because people were starving elsewhere in the world.

Of course, children should appreciate the value of food. It is appropriate to honor what it takes to procure food and to respect food by not wasting this critical resource that so many people lack. But while the statements made to you as a child were no doubt true (your parents probably *did* work hard to buy you those peas and carrots, and food *is* something for which we can feel gratitude and ideally avoid wasting, and people really *do* starve all over the world), ignoring what your body was telling you about being full did nothing to address these issues. What this perspective did, instead, was establish a link between guilt, obligation, and food. The price of membership in the Clean-Plate Club was learning to ignore inborn hunger and fullness cues.

Some people grow up feeling obligated to completely clean their plates. They carry old feelings of being disconnected from their hunger and fullness cues through adulthood. Many people raised with "Clean-Plate Club" rules even feel obligated to clear the plates of others. One of my earliest clients mentioned that she just could not allow herself to throw her children's leftover scraps away. She would eat what her kids wouldn't finish, whether she was particularly hungry or not.

When you make it a habit of eating whether or not you are hungry, you teach your body to disregard its own hunger and fullness cues. It is the ignoring of this innate feedback that leads to eating issues. Some people are so out of touch with their body's hunger or fullness signals that they are not even aware these cues exist. The truth is, ignoring fullness cues can lead to binging and discomfort from stuffing or overeating (this happens to many people at Thanksgiving). Ignoring hunger cues can lead to poor functioning and reduced concentration skills.

Self-Correction Toolkit for the Clean-Plate Eater

To gain the greatest benefit from this toolkit, I highly recommend you obtain a dedicated notebook to do your work in, or download our toolkit worksheets by visiting www.whydidijusteatthat.com/resources and click on the "Clean-Plate Eater" link for printable copies.

Belonging to the Clean-Plate Club encourages people to ignore their own Intuitive Eating instincts by basing their intake on visual cues (such as what is on the plate in front of them) rather than trusting their own internal hunger and fullness cues. Just as we can learn to finish everything on our plate, we can learn to listen to our bodies' fullness cues and stop eating when these cues tell us to.

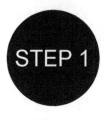

ADMIT...THEN COMMIT

Write a Starting-Point Affirmation

Admit that you understand, for your highest good, that there needs to be a change in your style of thinking. Take some quiet time to acknowledge this, then record your thoughts as an affirmation in your notebook or downloaded workbook pages: "I am releasing old 'shoulds' and ideas about food that no longer serve me. I am learning to become attuned to my body's cues about when I am hungry and when I am not. I am learning to honor these cues by not eating when I am not hungry." Then, sign and date it. I also recommend finding a moment to look in the mirror and tell yourself of this intention, and why—in your own words—it is important to you.

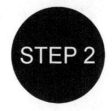

OBSERVE

You might take a moment to consider the food situation in your parents' past. Did they experience food insecurity? Did they experience famine or come from homes where food availability was uncertain? Were they raised by people who had these issues as children, resulting in these feelings spanning generations? It's important to understand your history and where the messages about eating and food that you got from your caregivers came from.

Think about how often you finish everything on your plate. Is this due to hunger? Or is it due to a sense of obligation to clean your plate?

NUTRITION BYTE: Letting go of "shoulds" is one simple but very powerful way to own our empowerment over our intake of food.

Food Diary Instructions

First, you'll need to become aware of your own hunger/fullness meter. Your hunger/fullness meter is a scale that measures the range of sensations from feeling hungry to feeling full in increments of 1 to 10, with "1" being super hungry and "10" feeling excessively full.

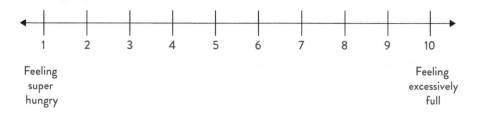

Food Diary

Once you are familiar with your hunger/fullness meter, keep a food diary for one week. Each diary page consists of three columns dividing the page length-wise. You can draw two vertical lines in your notebook, or use the downloaded worksheets.

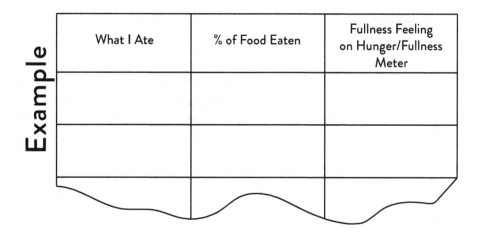

The first column describes what you ate, the second describes the percentage of food eaten on your plate, and the third describes when you stopped eating, and your feeling fullness on your hunger/fullness meter. I recommend people stop eating at around "7." (Ideally, "7" describes the point where you feel you've had enough to eat, but do not feel overly full.)

Make particular note of occasions when you ate out of feelings of obligation. These incidents might occur when you eat the last bit of food on your plate, even though you have the sense that you are no longer hungry and you don't particularly want to eat any more. Other incidents might include finishing uneaten food off of the plate of a partner or children in your care.

At the end of the week, what do you notice? Does finishing everything on your plate push you to a "9" or a "10," excessively full?

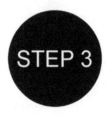

REWORK AND REFRAME

At the start of the following week, it's time to start a second set of worksheets, similar to the last one.

	Hunger/Full Scale at Start of Meal	Hunger/Full Scale at Middle of Meal	Hunger/Full Scale at End of Meal
Example			

This time, the worksheet will encourage you toward a mindful goal to stop eating at a level of around "7" on your hunger/fullness meter. Check in with your internal hunger/fullness rating before the meal, in the middle of the meal, and at the end of the meal. Where are you on a scale of 1 to 10 at each of these points? (The number you are at in the middle of a meal is very significant as it signals your brain and stomach just how far away you are from the meal ending and from you being full enough.)

If you find yourself feeling obligated to finish everything on your plate, a good solution to avoid leaving food uneaten is to simply give yourself smaller servings.

If you find yourself eating the uneaten food off of your kids' plates, smaller servings are an especially good idea. Hungry children tend to overestimate how much food they will be interested in eating before they hit the point when they are no longer hungry. Their eyes, as the expression goes, are often bigger than their stomachs.

Here's a handy tip: using smaller plates automatically forces us to take less food, cutting down on serving sizes. Remember, you can always go back for more if you have still not reached adequate fullness.

Some people eat leftovers because the bit of leftover food might seem too small to stick in a Pyrex container and put in the fridge, but too good to toss in the trash. In that case, why not get some smaller storage containers, or reuse small jelly jars? You can have them handy when you need a little snack later on, and can avoid eating something at a time you don't really want to eat.

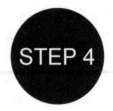

EMBRACE EATING INTUITIVELY

Eating Intuitively is governed by instinct and promotes listening to our own bodies. It lets our bodies decide when we are hungry and want to eat, and when we are full and it's time to stop eating. It's about just being in your body and learning to listen to what your body is telling you...not what your plate is saying.

If you have lost the capacity to "hear" these cues, you can regain the ability to do so by eating slowly and paying renewed, close attention to what your body is experiencing. Make it a habit to check in with you hunger/fullness cues regularly. You might even make a schedule of such check-ins, until the feelings show up without your looking for them. The more you practice focusing on your hunger/fullness meter, the more you will be able to develop your own emerging internal cues as a way to determine how much to eat, rather than simply eating whatever food ends up on the plate in front of you.

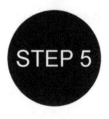

AFFIRM WHO YOU ARE

We began these exercises with a statement of acknowledgment, and we'll end with one, In your notebook or workbook, write down the following statement, putting your name in the provided blank space. This is an affirmation for you to repeat to yourself every day for at least a month, or whenever you feel obligated to finish the food on a plate when you are not hungry.

I am _____. I honor the wisdom of my body and pay attention to the cues that my body alerts me with. I eat when, hungry, stop when satisfied, and am grateful for my food.

3

THE LESS-MINDFUL EATER

I f you've ever sat in a movie theater munching away on popcorn while engrossed in some gripping drama, you've experienced automatic eating. We've all had the experience of being captivated by something on screen while absentmindedly popping food into our mouths, only to discover that we hadn't been paying attention to what we were eating at all. We're left thinking: "What happened? Everything I was eating is just about gone!"

I don't mean to say that enjoying an evening at the movies while holding a soft drink and a bag of popcorn isn't a perfectly fine way to have a good time. The problem emerges when, for some people, this so-called automatic eating becomes a habit in their everyday lives. For these people, it is commonplace to consume more food than intended. And in many cases, the meals themselves tend to be somewhat unbalanced; it is more likely that someone would automatically eat an overabundance of French fries than, say, salad.

THE LESS-MINDFUL EATER

The Less-Mindful Eater not only tends to be disconnected from what and how they eat, but also lacks the intuitive awareness of what types of food their body wants nutritionally. Moreover, they tend to be disconnected to times when their hunger has been satisfied. It is not unusual to find this person eating on a kind of autopilot, unconsciously consuming until they realize they feel overstuffed.

Twenty-eight-year-old Dwayne ran a small IT department at a large law firm; he found his job satisfying but extremely demanding. He usually had a difficult time waking up in the morning, and often rushed out of the house without breakfast, at most taking a cup of instant coffee in a to-go mug to drink in the car on the way to work. He didn't really have any sort of food plan for the day, which was usually super busy. The first meal he ate was lunch; he'd be so famished at that point he would eat more than he'd like to (usually while looking at his phone, barely aware he was eating). Sometimes he'd grab something from a vending machine for a pick-me-up later in the day.

By the time he left work (often after seven o'clock) he was again famished. He'd stop for fast food on his way home, which he ate mechanically while watching Netflix on his computer, always finishing it all because he'd be so distracted by whatever he was watching that he'd continue eating past the point where he was no longer hungry. Later, before he went to bed, he'd sometimes have a snack of something like popcorn, again while watching TV.

Dwayne came to my office wanting to eat healthier. He admitted to me that he had ADHD with a tendency to hyper-focus and that it was difficult for him to pay attention to anything that wasn't on task.

We discussed the possibility of starting meds for ADHD, but agreed to explore other strategies first. I suggested that by putting no effort into his meal planning and preparation, he had been demonstrating to himself that maintaining his health required less care than addressing the needs of his work. Part of the necessary shift he'd need to make would be to acknowledge that his own self-care was important. Since he was task-oriented, why not make healthy eating one of his daily tasks? I explained the value of planning the times and contents of meals a few days in advance of eating them.

Together, we created a structured daily schedule that included meals as part of the timeline. We planned a simple, loose menu that had three columns: one marked *Protein*, one marked *Starches*, and one marked *Fruits/Veggies*; he was to pick one item from each column for each meal. Dwayne committed to shopping Saturday mornings. Since he didn't enjoy cooking, he would buy pre-cooked chicken breasts, fish, turkey, etc., to freeze in portion-sized storage bags. He could thaw these foods by placing them in the fridge the night before use, along with frozen veggies and prepared rice or potatoes. He'd get enough food for seven dinners and seven breakfasts. Each weekend, he'd plan the menu for the following week.

Since mornings were difficult for him, it was best for him to do things like prep Wednesday's breakfast and dinner right after he finished eating Tuesday night's dinner. His breakfasts were small bites he could take to work and eat during morning breaks so he wouldn't be very hungry when lunch rolled around. He also agreed to stop snacking so close to bedtime, swapping the popcorn snack for an herbal tea he liked.

Most importantly, I suggested that he not look at screens while eating, so he could be more aware of the experience of enjoying his meal. This would allow him to have a deeper awareness of his body's fullness cue so he could stop eating when his appetite was satisfied.

After a couple of weeks, Dwayne reported eating more regularly and feeling more energetic. And although his primary goal was not to lose weight, he reported losing 20 pounds over the course of the year.

Self-Correction Toolkit for the Less-Mindful Eater

To gain the greatest benefit from this toolkit, I highly recommend you obtain a dedicated notebook to do your work in, or download our toolkit worksheets by visiting www.whydidijusteatthat.com/resources and click on the "Less-Mindful Eater" link for printable copies.

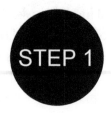

STEP 1

ADMIT...THEN COMMIT

Admit that you understand, for your highest good, that there needs to be a change in your approach to food and eating. Mechanical eaters tend to not prioritize food (and sometimes not prioritize other types of self-care as well). Take some quiet time to acknowledge this.

Write a Starting-Point Affirmation

You might write down something like, "I am opening myself up to being more present and accepting increasing awareness of what my body is experiencing and what it needs, especially around eating and food," in the space marked Affirmations below, then sign and date it. I also recommend finding a moment to look in the mirror and tell yourself this intention and to explain why—in your own words—this is important to you.

NUTRITION BYTE: When you commit to being aware of what your body is feeling, you become more aware of you own hunger and fullness cues. As you allow these cues to grow more noticeable, they become signals from your body: telling you when it wants to start eating, and when it wants to stop eating.

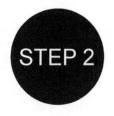

OBSERVE

The first step toward positive change is the simple act of observation. Observing instances of not being mindful around food may not be easy for people who have become used to not paying attention, at least at first. So do your best and allow yourself as steep a learning curve as you might need.

As is the case with a few other people working to shift their eating styles, I recommend keeping a diary of your day so you can track what you eat. If you find yourself being unmindful regarding other aspects of your personal habits that result in poor self-care, you might want to track those elements too.

An out-of-balance food diary (that reflects inadequate nutrition) might look something like this:

Example of an inadvisable, Out-of-Balance Eating Schedule

Ex**a**m**p**l**e**	7:10	Coffee with milk
	8:07	Bagel and cream cheese
	9:12	Yogurt
	10:00	5 crackers
	10:32	2 small cookies
	11:39	2 cheese sticks
	12:30	Apple and potato chips
	2:00	Sliced turkey
	4:37	Salted nuts
	6:45	Frozen dinner (chicken, broccoli, rice)
	7:31	1/2 grilled cheese sandwich
	8:35	Ice cream and cookies

If you have the sense that—up until now—your eating has been unbalanced, fear not! In our next step, we'll discuss a helpful way forward.

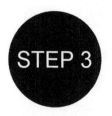

STEP 3

REFRAME A MINDFUL RELATIONSHIP WITH FOOD

The purpose of this step is to help you shift your relationship with food from indifference to proactive awareness, so that eventually your mindful approach becomes an every-day conscious habit of being.

There is a two-part exercise I recommend to help people become more mindful as eaters. This step is critical because bringing mindfulness to one's relationship with food invites a deeper sense of gratitude, which in turn encourages more joy and satisfaction, not to mention healthy portion control.

Activity: Mindful Bites

PART ONE:

You'll need a raisin.

We recommend raisins because they're small, unremarkable, and most people can take 'em or leave 'em. Not the type of food that usually commands our full attention, but it is our full attention we are actually going to bring to this little shriveled grape. So...once you have your raisin, we'll move forward

1. First, hold your raisin up to your eyes and get a good look at it. Notice its shape, its color, its wrinkled texture.
2. Next, see if it has a distinct smell. Give it a gentle squeeze; is it plump with a little flexible "give" or is it a bit dry and somewhat rigid? Give it a lick. How does it feel on your tongue?
3. Then slowly bite it, and feel your teeth break through the raisin, paying attention to that sensation.
4. And finally, thoughtfully chew the raisin, and taste it. Consider the flavor. Is it tasty, or so-so, or unpleasant? Does it remind you of any other foods? How does it feel in your mouth?
5. After you've finished eating your raisin, consider the fact that it was once a grape on a vine on a farm that required people to harvest and dry and pack and get to the market where you acquired it among a whole bunch of other raisins. Perhaps you might have a moment of gratitude for the miracle of nature that created the raisin as well as for the human labor that got the raisin to you, including money you earned to purchase the raisin.

PART TWO:

The next part of the Mindful Bite exercise is pretty much the same as the first part, only this time you can repeat the steps of the raisin process with a bit of food that would be a treat for you, maybe one that you would typically eat, bite after bite, without much thought. This bit of food might be a cookie or a piece of fruit or a French fry or a piece of sushi... anything, as long as it's something you enjoy.

Repeat the above five steps with this item. After you've paid close sensory attention to your "Part Two" sample, take a moment to reflect on your experience. Consider your sense of satisfaction with that food in the aftermath of your ultra-mindful enjoyment of it. How has consuming it slowly and with care changed your experience of eating? Has your relationship with this particular food itself changed?

Of course, it is not practical to treat every bite of food you eat in this time-consuming manner, but I do recommend you run through this exercise—or at least an abbreviated version if time does not permit—on the first bite of each meal every day for a week, as part of the new habit you'll begin to implement. We'll discuss this new habit in Step Four.

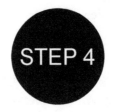

IMPLEMENTING NEW HABITS

Step Three communicated the idea that enjoying and appreciating food is more than just biting, chewing, and swallowing. Your new mindful, more self-aware way of eating is even more powerful and useful when you give this approach a defined schedule. I find that it is helpful to have a structured plan for your eating, though it is fine to be flexible with the demands of the day. (Dwayne, whose experience we discussed earlier in the chapter, programmed his schedule as reminder alarms in his Google calendar.)

Using the following worksheet as a model, create your own schedule of positive eating and related self-care choices. (Ideally, the meals/snacks should be balanced, consisting of proteins, starches, and fruits and veggies. Snacks should be likewise varied: fruit, nuts, carrots and humus, etc.)

Example of Implementing New Habits Schedule

Example	7:10–7:30	Wake up
	7:30–8:30	Breakfast (Remember to Enjoy A First Mindful Bite!)
	10:00–10:30	Snack (Remember to Enjoy A First Mindful Bite!)
	12:30–1:00	Lunch (Remember to Enjoy A First Mindful Bite!)
	3:00–3:30	Snack (Remember to Enjoy A First Mindful Bite!)
	6:00–6:30	Dinner (Remember to Enjoy A First Mindful Bite!)
	8:30–9:00	Optional small snack (Remember to Enjoy A First Mindful Bite!)
	11:00–11:30	Bedtime

And now it's your turn! Create a nutrition schedule table in your notebook, or download the Nutrition Schedule workbook pages from the Less Mindful Eater document in this book's online resource pages. If you are creating a schedule in your notebook, create the table in half-hour intervals. You do not need to write anything in every space, but everyone's schedule is different, and we want to allow for flexibility.

A final note: Many people multitask due to a perceived lack of time and find themselves doing things like eating a sandwich while working at their desk. I would imagine that in many cases these people could honor themselves with a mindfulness break over the few minutes it takes to eat that sandwich. In situations like this, I'd suggest that if you must eat in front of the computer, at least minimize your work screens (and video screens, news reports, game screens, etc.) or anything that demands your attention. Put on music you find introspective and eat mindfully, aware of the taste and sensations of eating (and hopefully enjoying) your sandwich. Of course, the additional bonus of taking a moment to enjoy a mindful bite at the start is always a great idea!

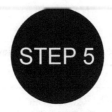

AFFIRM WHO YOU ARE

We opened these exercises with one affirmation, and we will close them with another. This final step is an ongoing process to take firm ownership of a more flexible way of interacting with your world.

In your notebook or workbook, write down the following statement, putting your name in the provided blank space.:

> I am _____. My heart is open, my attitude is flexible, and I mindfully enjoy my food with gratitude while being fully present.

Celebrate and take ownership of your new mindful approach! Repeat your affirmation every day. If you forget, that's fine, just forgive yourself and pick up where you left off. Even if you don't fully believe this statement at first, remember that in order to grow, we must become clear on what we aspire to be

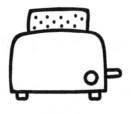

4

THE LESS-STRUCTURED EATER

For the most part, structure is an important part of our lives. During the week, when we're either at school or at work, our days are usually structured. We wake up at a certain time, we go to school or work at a certain time, and we have breaks that are set at certain times. Most people will say that this type of structure allows them to eat in a more balanced, mindful way during the day, though that is not necessarily true for everyone. Many people have no rhyme or reason to their eating habits, despite operating within a daily schedule.

The evenings can be particularly tough for many people as that time of day often provides less external structure. After a long day when we get home and have free time, food can be a way to unwind or to reward ourselves for working hard. Many of us are tired and stressed and often reach for food as a way of vegging or numbing out. Similarly, on weekends or when we're on vacation, our time is much less structured, making it even more difficult for people to eat in a nourishing, balanced way.

THE LESS-STRUCTURED EATER

When I asked Kavitha—a 39-year-old sales rep and mother of three—to describe what her eating looked like on a typical day, her first reaction was a sort of blank stare. It was as if she didn't understand the words I was saying. After a little while, she guessed that there hadn't been any structure or consistency to her eating in years, musing, "I'm what I'd call a *professional grazer.*"

She went on to say that she didn't eat structured meals or snacks, but instead would simply grab food whenever she felt the whim. When she prepared dinner or packed school lunches for her kids, she'd nibble at what she was preparing, but rarely sat down to properly eat. When I asked if she was hungry at the times she did stop to eat, she shrugged indifferently, claiming, "I'm never hungry. I don't allow myself to get there." I asked her whether she took time at these "grazing breaks" to stop and be present while she ate. She told me that she usually grabbed her food while doing something else, like checking work orders or, at the very least, checking out Facebook on her phone.

The first thing we did was build some nutrition structure into her day. We drew up a schedule consisting of three meals with planned snacks in between. I asked her to sit down when she ate and do nothing aside from eating. I suggested she take time to observe the practice of eating, noticing the taste and texture of what she was consuming.

This approach felt so odd to her that she actually needed to set the timer on her watch as a reminder to eat. Since we had limited her multiple (but scattershot) snack times to an organized few, she had the opportunity to begin to be aware of and work with the sensation of being hungry. In subsequent sessions, as she understood how hunger and fullness cues helped her regulate healthy nutrition eating habits, she was able to rely on hunger and fullness cues to determine meal or snack size. And as she felt herself become more present at meal and snack times, this mindful approach helped make sure she was not eating more than she actually wanted.

Self-Correction Toolkit for the Less-Structured Eater

> To gain the greatest benefit from this toolkit, I highly recommend you obtain a dedicated notebook to do your work in, or download our toolkit worksheets by visiting www.whydidijusteatthat.com/resources and click on the "Less-Structured Eater" link for printable copies.

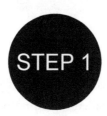

ADMIT...THEN COMMIT

To start off, admit that you understand, for your highest good, that there needs to be a change in your way of doing things. Lack of structure may seem freeing, but in reality it creates its own repression by setting up more challenges than having reasonable structures in place would.

Write a Starting-Point Affirmation

Boundaries may feel like restrictions, but their highest contribution is that they define our self-care best-practices. Take some quiet time to acknowledge this, then record your thoughts in your notebook or the downloaded workbook pages. You might write down, "I am creating more structure to best serve my life and eating habits," in the space marked Affirmations below, then sign and date it. I also recommend finding a moment to look in the mirror and tell yourself this intention, and why—in your own words— it is important to you.

NUTRITION BYTE: Taking time to be prepared is prime self-care in action; it's easier to achieve goals with a strategy in place and all relevant elements ready for use.

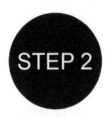

STEP 2

OBSERVE

Keep a food diary for three days, eating as you have been doing up until now. Take care to be very detailed regarding when and what you are eating day to day. Create a food diary table in your notebook, or download the food diary workbook pages from the Less-Structured Eater document in this book's online resource pages. If you are creating a schedule in your notebook, create the table in half-hour intervals, allowing space for three columns to include three days' worth of information (partial example layout below). Include every snack, cup of coffee, and muffin eaten on the run.

	Time	Day One	Day Two	Day Three
Example	7:00-7:30			
	7:30-8:00			
	8:00-8:30			

When you've completed the chart following the third day, assess the information. Do you notice when you are eating full, balanced meals, and when you are not? Are you starving yourself early in the day only to over-consume toward the end? Are you making healthy and wholesome choices that can help you function at your best all day, or do you find yourself "running on fumes" for periods of time? What else have you noticed?

Write your observations on the pages following the diary.

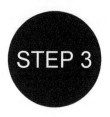

REWORK AND REFRAME

A structured daily schedule helps to create a structured eating plan; building structure is very important. On days when there is no school or work it can be helpful if you create an hourly schedule. By creating a schedule, you're much more likely to get things done. In addition to completing tasks, you're more likely to be able to follow through with meals and snacks that are planned for specific times. It is especially helpful to plan out the contents of the meals and snacks in advance, along with the times.

The solution here is to plan out your menu in advance to make sure that you have available the foods that you want, when you want. Many of my clients like to meal prep on the weekends when they have more time. They wrap up food into smaller portions and freeze it. Each night, they take a portion out of the freezer and put it in the fridge so that it's mostly defrosted by the time they're ready to eat dinner the following day. This requires some planning and forethought.

Giving yourself permission to eat a wide variety of foods is crucial here!

Worksheet

Utilize a chart where you can plan your day and schedule your time. You can create a food diary table in your notebook, or download the food diary workbook pages from the Less-Structured Eater document in this book's online resource pages. If you are creating a schedule in your note-book, create the table in half-hour intervals, with a column setting times and a column listing meals and snacks in your schedule, (example layout below.)

Try to be specific with your plan for the evening, as for most this is the hardest time of the day. Feel free to set the specific meal and snack times to suit your activity schedule, making sure to remain mindful of the recommended intervals between eating times.

	Time	Meal
E x a m p l e	7:00-7:30	
	7:30-8:00	
	8:00-8:30	

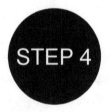

STEP 4

COMMITTING TO NEW BEHAVIORS

This exercise is an important step in creating lasting and meaningful change. For many who are not used to having a firm schedule, the abrupt imposition of structure might bring up some feelings of resistance. This is a completely natural response. After all, who enjoys being pushed out of their comfort zone?

So if any thoughts of anger, resentment, resistance or negativity show up, have a conversation with yourself. For example, you might write down something like:

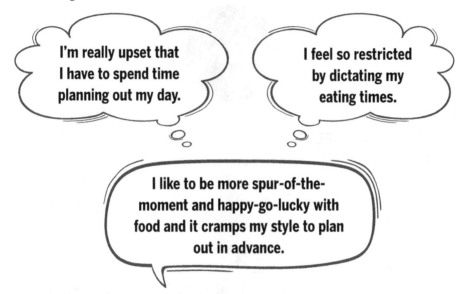

And then answer your concern with a constructive response, something like:

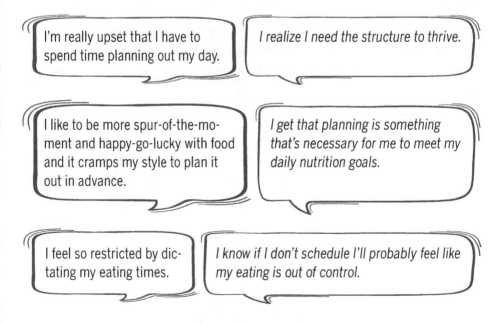

**Now it is your turn to have the conversation
in your own notebook or workbook pages...**

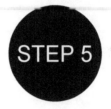

AFFIRM WHO YOU ARE

Finally, lock in your new and evolved approach by making this statement your own. We opened these exercises with one affirmation, and we will close them with another. This final step is an ongoing process to take firm ownership of a more flexible way of interacting with your world.

In your notebook or workbook, write down the following statement, putting your name in the provided blank space.:

Now repeat the phrase below, filling in the blank with your name and other words:

> I am _____. My heart is open, my attitude is flexible, and I gratefully accept and follow through on the planning and organization steps appropriate for making life better for me and those in my world.

It's a good idea to say your affirmation to yourself each morning. (Make it part of your schedule!) You might also say it to yourself in those moments when you feel a bit challenged by following your new daily schedule.

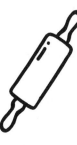

5

THE FAD-FOOD EATER

For at least a hundred years, the for-profit diet industry has pushed fad diets and quick shortcuts guaranteeing you health and the "perfect body." These fad diets are promoted by a mixture of self-proclaimed "experts," brick-and-mortar institutions and franchises, and media-propelled influencers. Often, people with no formal nutrition training sell themselves as health or weight-loss coaches. Modern "diet culture" includes not only the diet industry, but all of the consumers who buy into the ideas that the industry puts forth. Under its influence, too many eating approaches are advertised without much scientific or mental health expertise, and too many people unquestioningly adopt these approaches.

How many fad diets have you been on? I have to admit that when I was a kid growing up in suburban New York, I was on a few of these iffy diets myself! But if something seems too good to be true, it probably is.

THE FAD-FOOD EATER

Many people find highly structured diets (that leave little room for choice and dictate strict eating rules) extremely appealing. They choose to go on restrictive diets because they feel like something is out of control about their eating...but by applying harsh constraints, they only gain an illusion of order while the diet actually knocks their relationship with food (as well as their metabolism) even more out of balance.

What we have long known about fad diets is that they're not sustainable in the long run. Going on and off fad diets (also known as yo-yo dieting) almost always results in the opposite of what was intended. Diets promoting sudden, drastic changes only work for a comparatively minuscule number of dieters. Ironically enough, the complete opposite approach often works best: making small, incremental changes over an extended period is most effective for meaningful change.

Fads are not merely limited to diets alone. Not long after I began working on this book, I happened to go out to dinner with a friend. She wasn't a client, but she said something that reflects an issue shared by many people I see in my consultation room. We were ordering salads, and I had decided on a mixed kale dish. At my choice, my friend looked a little shocked.

"Haven't you heard," she asked with surprise, "that kale is out and watercress is in?"

The truth was that I had eaten watercress just the day before, but I like to rotate my food intake, since each different food item has nutrients in its own, unique way and I believe in getting as wide a variety of nutrition as possible. The idea that some foods are suddenly "in" while others are suddenly "out" has a lot to do with magazine and blog writers needing material to write about. They often seize upon a new scientific study, pluck a new factoid from it, and fling it into some media outlet. While there is a lot of good nutrition journalism at your fingertips, there is a whole lot of misinterpreted and incomplete information readily available as well. And because of that, my friend bought into that unhelpful tendency many people have to sort foods into "good" foods and "bad" foods—categories that are ever-shifting based on the latest lifestyle report.

There is something resembling a non-stop drumbeat of media in our lives, both internet-based and traditional. Magazines, websites, TV news reports...what seems like countless content-providers looking for fresh, compelling information to attract eyeballs. In our food-obsessed culture, it should come as no surprise that there is a stream of information, breathless and enthusiastic, about the latest news that is sure to be replaced by something else just as earthshaking in the coming days or weeks. Some of the stuff they report has value, while some of it is pure nonsense. Either way, strictly following this information is no way to form an eating strategy.

For example: In the (current as I write these words) debate between kale vs. watercress, watercress had been established as chock-full of valuable nutrients while, on the kale side, some concerns had been raised regarding the downside of eating mega-amounts of that vegetable. The truth is, I believe that we should eat as much variety as possible, and that mega-amounts of anything is probably not a great idea.

Diets or otherwise, the danger of fad eating is two-fold. Nutrition advice found online and in magazine blurbs is frequently incomplete and subject to change; and this change is often in the form of completely contradictory follow-up information. People who follow fads too closely tend to go from one restrictive eating plan to another restrictive eating plan, exchanging the joy in eating for judgment and inflexibility. Moreover, in the blizzard of information, people can get inundated with context-less facts. At a certain point, they give up trying to eat healthfully because so much of what's out there negates itself. They can't trust what's healthy anyway, so they surrender to eating without any sort of discernment at all.

Fad hopping can even —in some cases —lead to orthorexia, where in an effort to avoid all the so-called "bad" foods, people limit their diets to the point that they are not properly nourished.

In most cases, unless you are getting specific instructions by a healthcare provider with expertise in diet and nutrition, do not plan your meal choices based on diet fads and trendy "shoulds." I counsel people to take advantage of the wide range of wholesome foods they can access, and to not get bound up in the latest craze.

Self-Correction Toolkit for the Fad-Food Eater

> To gain the greatest benefit from this toolkit, I highly recommend you obtain a dedicated notebook to do your work in, or download our toolkit worksheets by visiting www.whydidijusteatthat.com/resources and click on the "Fad-Food Eater" link for printable copies.

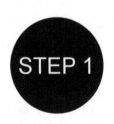

STEP 1

ADMIT...THEN COMMIT

In my consultation office, I often speak with clients who are tired of jumping from diet to diet—each diet selling a different approach. It seems that almost everyone is at least somewhat bewildered by the blizzard of often contradictory nutrition and diet information that comes our way. "I give up," is a-not-uncommon phrase I hear.

And momentarily giving up may not be such a bad thing. To surrender aspects of the past and admit we're ready for change can be a really constructive choice. So for Step One, take some quiet time to acknowledge a commitment to a new and healthy relationship with food, one not restricted by shoulds/shouldn'ts and the latest fads.

Write a Starting-Point Affirmation

Admit that you understand, for your highest good, that there needs to be a change in your style of thinking. Take some quiet time to acknowledge this, then record your thoughts in your notebook or the downloaded workbook pages. You might write, "I am flexible in my approach to food. I honor my body, trusting its intuition by eating a wide variety of nutritious foods when I am hungry (and working in some 'fun foods' too!) and stopping when I am no longer hungry." Then sign and date it. I also recommend finding a moment each day to look in the mirror and remind yourself of this intention, and why—in your own words—this is important to you.

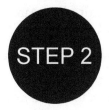

OBSERVE

I'm going to give you some homework. Don't worry, the deadline is completely up to you, and it won't be graded. But it is important.

To the best of your recollection, make a list of the various diets you've ever been on, and the approximate dates and durations. Memory can be unreliable at first, especially when it comes to plans that did not work out as hoped for. So it may take you a little while to fully complete this exercise, and that's okay. It is important to take stock of where you are coming from, in order to help frame the direction you wish to go in.

As you make your list, make note of a few important elements:

Where did you first hear of each diet? Were the sources reliable, or something a bit more shaky? Perhaps you read about it online or in a magazine? How did you feel at the start of the diet? How did you feel at the end? Why did this way of eating end? Are you pleased with the outcome of any of these diets? Knowing what you know now, would you have embarked on any of them in the first place?

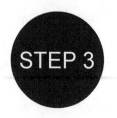

CHALLENGING OLD BEHAVIORS

After you have completed the first section, here are a few more things to consider about your current attitude toward dieting:

Additional Questions:

Do you feel you must have restrictions attached to your eating or you might lose control?

Do you feel like you have a love/hate relationship with the idea of conventional restrictive dieting?

What have you learned about yourself when it comes to dieting?

Do you feel that conventional restrictive dieting works for you?

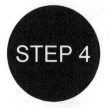

NEW DIRECTIONS

What we call diets—be they fad diets, medical diets or religious diets— are really just *eating strategies*. I would never suggest people replace a diet (even a diet I would consider problematic) with no eating strategy at all.

My guidance is for people to acknowledge that adapting an eating strategy is important; what matters is what that strategy is, and how it works. So rather than back into yet another eating strategy based on fad thinking, I suggest you first give some thought to how a new empowering, healthy eating strategy might manifest.

- What would your ideal strategy look like?

- What benefits of a new eating strategy do you wish to have?
- How would a positive, new eating strategy affect not only your eating habits but how you perceive yourself?

I've long maintained that changing our relationships with food is tied to changing our relationships with ourselves. You simply cannot change one without changing the other. So the first step to changing both of these relationships is to embrace mindfulness.

Take time to be aware of what you are experiencing moment to moment. Pay attention to whatever feelings of gratitude you hold for whatever experiences you feel grateful for. Especially focus on what your body is experiencing and feeling.

As you become more cognizant of what your body is feeling, you cannot help but become more aware of your own sense of hunger and fullness. You may feel these right away, or it may take some time to reconnect with these feelings, but stick with it. As your hunger and fullness cues become more present, they can become the signals that determine when you start eating, and when you stop eating.

A helpful way to look at this is to think in terms of your "hunger/fullness meter," a scale that measures the range of sensations from feeling hungry to feeling full in increments of 1 to 10, with "1" being super hungry and "10" being excessively full.

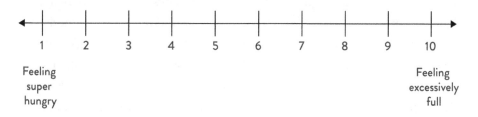

A way to connect with this important aspect of listening to your body is to keep track of what you eat as it relates to your hunger/fullness sensations.

A targeted diary can be very helpful in this area, which you can create in your notebook, or by downloading the food diary workbook pages from the Food Fad Eater pages document in this book's online resource section. If you are creating a schedule in your notebook, create the table by day and time, by hunger and fullness levels, and by meals and snacks. (See the illustration below.) Filling in the information at each meal is an effective way to get a sense of how attuned you are with your body's cues. (I recommend that people try not to let their hunger drop below "3," and that they stop eating at around "7.")

	Day/ Time	Hunger level	Breakfast	Optional Snack	Lunch	Optional Snack	Dinner	Optional Snack
Example								

The approach of following your body's hunger/fullness cues makes it easy to let go of the rule-based approach of dieting, allowing you to decide "how much" to eat. But diet-induced deprivation includes a lot more than simply ignoring how much your body needs. It is also about denying foods you might like, but consider "bad." (As I frequently point out, I don't consider any food to be a "bad food" unless it is actually toxic, moldy, stale, rotten, or triggers adverse allergic reactions.) I believe there are nutritionally dense foods that are good to organize your meals around, and other foods that are less nutritionally dense and best eaten as less-frequent treats. But that does not mean that these treat foods should be avoided at all costs. In fact, a major benefit of eating intuitively is that it releases us from that frustrating conflict we experience with foods we want to eat but feel that we're "not allowed" to.

The core of the "not allowed to" restriction is disempowerment. (For example, saying "I want to eat ice cream, but I'm not allowed to" can also be read as, "I want to eat ice cream, but I'm not empowered to eat the things I want.") At the very least, this dynamic is unpleasant. At the very worst, it is difficult to maintain. Consider, then, how empowering is the concept of, "I am empowered to eat ice cream, but I choose not to at this moment." It puts the power to eat ice cream—or not to eat ice cream—under your control.

Now let's take this idea a little further. In a conventional diet, a person's inner dialogue—slightly exaggerated to make the point—might go like this, as they were offered a piece of chocolate cake, and turned it down:

> *"Oooh! Chocolate cake for dessert. Boy, I do like chocolate cake. But I can't eat cake. The rules of this diet say no chocolate cake. So I won't have some. Aw, but it looks so good. No, I really shouldn't. I really want some, but I can't have any. Ugh! Darn it!"*

Or sometimes, the outcome looks like this: *"I ate it anyway and now I'm beating myself up."*

Perhaps in reading about the person turning down the cake, you felt frustrated and got a sense of the sacrifice they were feeling, and even a tinge of their resentment. Or in the case of the person eating the cake and then regretting it, you sympathized with their sense of shame.

But now, let's imagine the inner dialogue—slightly exaggerated again, to make the point—of someone instinctual eating approach as they were offered a piece of chocolate cake that they turned down:

> *"Oooh! Chocolate cake for dessert. Boy, I do like chocolate cake. And I can have a slice now if I really want it. But do I want a slice? How will I feel if I eat it now? I can always have one tomorrow if I want. Or next week. Or next month. Or whenever, because when I decide to have chocolate cake, it's my choice. At this particular moment I feel pretty full from*

dinner. So I think I'll pass tonight, and have some another time, when I really want it."

See how turning down the cake in this instance was actually an empowering experience?

Of course, our intuitive eater in this scenario could have just as easily had a piece, or maybe a small taste, and that would have been fine, too. Because as they listen to what their body wants, they will tend to follow eating approaches that might not be perfect, but are good enough. After all, eating intuitively is all about flexibility. With just a shift in attitude, it becomes easier for most people to stick to a balanced approach, instead of restrictive diets.

(I should note here that there is more to making positive eating choices than embracing mindfulness. Balanced eating choices are based on more than one aspect, including understanding sound nutrition principles and one's relationship with food. This book is primarily focused on approaches to improving one's relationship with food. Sound nutrition principles—like eating a varied diet high in vegetables—become easier to follow when one's emotional relationship with food is healthy.)

An approach called intuitive eating—which has been growing in popularity since its emergence in the 1990s—has been teaching people to relax their stringent attitudes toward food and eating. Intuition, after all, is governed by instinct, not rules, and so intuitive eating rejects rule-based diets in favor of listening to one's own body. Intuitive eating lets our bodies decide when we are hungry and want to eat, and when we are full and it's time to stop eating. It discards the "shoulds" of restrictive diets (you *should* eat this, you *should not* eat that) in favor of a "good enough is actually, well, good enough" approach. It removes all stigmas and self-contempt from your relationship with food and eating. It is less about rules and more about a way of being. If there are no rules, there is nothing to violate and nothing to beat yourself up over. It's about just you being you in your body, and learning to listen to what your body is telling you. It actively encourages a positive relationship with food and eating. The whole point of food, after all, is enjoyment, satisfaction and nourishment.

It may take a little while to retrain yourself away from the old inflexible diet rules and restrictions you used to follow, but trust the wisdom of your body! The changes offered by the intuitive eating strategy are not as drastic—or as unrealistic —as the results that fad and crash diets claim, but over time people do achieve positive and healthy long-term outcomes.

NUTRITION BYTE: Intuitive Eating is an evidence-based framework and approach that rejects diet culture and the diet mentality. It views all foods as neutral and focuses on being attuned to the body's internal cues to allow the eater to make choices that feel right for them. It was developed by dietitians Elyse Resch and Evelyn Tribole in their 1995 book, *Intuitive Eating: A Revolutionary Program That Works,* and has continued through the fourth edition in 2020.

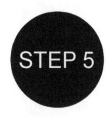

STEP 5

AFFIRM WHO YOU ARE

We began these exercises with a statement of acknowledgement, and we'll end with an affirmation for you to repeat to yourself every day for at least a month—at each meal, if necessary—or whenever you feel the urge to restrict your food in drastic ways. In your notebook or workbook, write down the following statement, putting your name in the provided blank space.:

I am_____. I honor the hunger and fullness cues that my body uses to alert me. I eat when hungry and stop when satisfied. I can eat treats I enjoy or I can put these foods aside for another time, because I am an empowered eater.

If you forget to say your affirmation now and then, that's fine; just forgive yourself and pick up where you left off. Even if you don't fully believe this statement at first, remember that in order to grow, we must become clear on what we aspire to be.

6

THE FOOD CUDDLER

For some people, food serves as a major source of comfort. It is not unusual for people growing up in households with a lot of anxiety or feelings of judgment and criticism to internalize the negativity of their surroundings. The options children have in processing emotional challenges is pretty limited, and many find comfort in food (for some of the reasons we've discussed in the first part of this book.) As they grow into adulthood, this sense of drawing comfort from food stays with them.

THE FOOD CUDDLER

Annamaria was a 47-year-old widow who realized that her eating habits had been interfering with her life and well-being for years. After the sudden, tragic loss of her husband in her early forties, Annamaria found comfort in food. Food, in fact, had claimed an important place in her life, beginning to serve as a substitute for love, companionship, and happiness. It was as though the feeling of fullness after eating a large meal or snack was giving her, as she described it, "a big hug from within." She used food as a way to numb the pain she was feeling. Eating eventually played such a central role in her life that she began to isolate herself from others. A heart-to-heart talk with an old high school friend brought about the realization for Annamaria that the time was right for change. At long last, she was ready to establish healthier, more constructive coping skills in which to channel her grief.

Looking back at her self-reported history, we discovered that Annamaria had actually grown up using food as a coping skill; it was the answer to making her feel better when she was a child. If she were upset, her mom would provide a plate of warm chocolate chip cookies and a glass of milk and would console her by saying, "Eat this and you will feel better." That message remained with her and became almost a guiding principle by which she lived. In addition to soothing childhood disappointments, food treats were also used as rewards for achievements in school or extracurricular activities like sports or music recitals. So, if Annamaria found eating to be a comforting tool toward getting past disappointments—perhaps as in that time she dealt with a disappointing high school crush when she was a teen—of course food would weigh heavily in dealing with more significant personal tragedies such as losing a spouse.

While habits established throughout a lifetime are by no means easily dismantled overnight, Annamaria's simply becoming aware of her emotion-triggered eating dynamics was an important first step toward healing her relationship with food. Understanding why she chose certain foods for comfort played a crucial role in starting to be able to make other choices to self-soothe. We put in place non-food strategies she might use when uncomfortable feelings arose. Over time, instead of using food to provide the comfort she craved, she was often able to stop and ask herself what it was that she really needed at any given moment. Of course, transcending food issues is an ongoing process, but over time Annamaria reports having a greater sense of control over food...instead of the other way around.

Food is certainly a source of love and warmth for many of us. Certain kinds of food might touch a warm spot in our hearts that bring back warm memories of sitting with a loving caregiver who offered comfort in a plate of warm chocolate chip cookies and a glass of milk. The downside, of course, is that too much reliance on food for comfort creates a skewed relationship with food and eating. This leads to troubling habits, especially when emotions are triggered by longstanding negative feelings.

Self-Correction Toolkit for the Food Cuddler

To gain the greatest benefit from this toolkit, I highly recommend you obtain a dedicated notebook to do your work in, or download our toolkit worksheets by visiting www.whydidijusteatthat.com/resources and click on the "Food Cuddler" link for printable copies.

Some of the fallout of negativity from the past lingers on as unaddressed habits stemming from deeply ingrained trauma. While it's unlikely we can completely get rid of all of whatever negative experiences or messages we were subjected to as children, we can at least learn to quiet down our hurt inner chatter so we can hear our more self-empowered mindset.

No matter what the level of childhood trauma was, when it becomes enmeshed with food being used as a soothing mechanism, resolving the eating issue can be particularly difficult to change. But with work and dedication, we might move mountains.

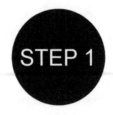

STEP 1

ADMIT...THEN COMMIT

Write a Starting-Point Affirmation

Admit that you understand, for your highest good, that there needs to be a change in your style of thinking. Take some quiet time to acknowledge this, then record your thoughts in your notebook or the downloaded workbook pages. You might write down, "I am learning to manage my stress with grace and flexibility, and soothing myself in ways that do not include food. I am committed to listening to my body's cues about when I am hungry and when I am not," then sign and date it. I also recommend finding a moment to look in the mirror and tell yourself of this intention, and why—in your own words—that this is important to you.

> **NUTRITION BYTE:** Our agitated emotional triggers can be louder than our body's intuitive hunger/fullness cues. So if we feel upset that we were triggered to eat in a way we really didn't want to, let's give ourselves a break—when we regain our emotional balance we can start back with intuition-based eating again!

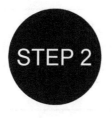

OBSERVE

Let's at first acknowledge that the impulse to eat is generally triggered by one of two kinds of motivations. The first kind is based on hunger cues elicited by the body's physical needs. The other kind stems from emotions or old behavioral triggers. Many people eat from a combination of both impulses and find themselves eating more than they'd like—or is particularly good for them—when the impulse is triggered by emotions, separate from physical feelings of actual hunger.

So, the first exercise is to take some time becoming mindful about when you eat. How much of it is due to feeling hungry, and how much of it is due to other, non-physical feelings?

Activity: Keep a Mood/Food Diary

Create a Mood/Food Diary in your notebook, or download the Mood/Food Diary workbook pages from the Food Cuddler document in this book's online resource pages. (See sample diary fragment below.)

Example

Date/Time	Food Consumed	Emotions/Triggers
Monday, 11:15AM	Leftover pasta, Half bowl	Feeling frustrated over fight with sister
Tuesday, 7:30PM	Container of ice cream	Stress with work project

Track everything you eat, and the corresponding mood for a week. Notice how often you go to use food because you are feeling upset, frustrated, or experiencing any similar negative emotions. Pay attention to between-meal snacks, as well as meals where you realize you are continuing to eat even after you are no longer hungry because you are feeling some level of emotional distress. These feelings may be very conspicuous, or they may be on the subtle side. Do your best to focus your awareness on whatever emotions you experience.

Though I recommend you follow this exercise for a week, continue to keep your diary until you are able to discern what you are feeling even as you feel triggered to eat. (At this point you are just observing, so do not feel the need to start to take any corrective actions just yet.)

And here's a twist: as time goes on, try to make a note of what you are feeling triggered by *before* you eat something.

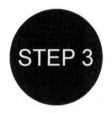

STEP 3

DISCOVERING NEW COMFORT STRATEGIES

Do you notice any patterns in your Mood/Food Diary? Did the additional awareness that you focused on your eating choices make the triggers more obvious to you? As you were maintaining your diary, were there certain patterns of emotion-triggers appearing in your notations?

Some emotion-triggers are rooted in direct experiences we have had earlier in our lives. For example, having someone make negative comments about your weight or appearance, (or having a parent who is angry about their own inability to control their weight, and projected that anger on you) is bound to create ongoing issues.

It really doesn't matter where, how, or even when the initial trauma occurred. Some people may not even be aware that there is significant trauma in their past because the trauma did not strike them directly. I often start by asking people to look back at their family system. We know anxiety is often passed down through genetic lines. Perhaps a not-too-distant ancestor's family was victimized by war, or perhaps illness created an orphan situation. While it is helpful to understand your individual family's trauma story, not everyone has access to that information. Many members of persecuted racial or ethnic groups may never know the specific details of their inherited trauma. What matters is that we take steps to let go of the emotional challenges that were rooted in the past while learning new ways to self-soothe in the present.

As you settled into the diary-keeping process, you (ideally) have started becoming somewhat more aware of your emotion triggers. Let's keep these identified triggers in mind as we move on to the next activity.

Some of your emotion triggers can be addressed directly. What I mean by that is that if you notice emotions reacting to specific triggers that you feel are no longer accurate or reflect who you really are, write down correc-tive thoughts. For example, you might have had an issue in high school that still kind of bothers you...even though it's been years since you were in high school and this specific issue no longer reflects who you are. If that is the case for you, you are being haunted by unpleasant echoes, not by any-thing in your current reality.

Activity: Create Statements That Release Negative Self-Talk

Make a list of any unpleasant echoes, and by each one create a statement that refutes them. Suppose, for instance, you saw yourself as painfully awk-ward in high school. On your list, you might write down something like, "Day by day I am becoming graceful and self-assured."

Release these wrong-headed triggers and let them out of your life!

Other emotion triggers can also be addressed indirectly. What I mean by that is there are ways to soothe yourself even in the face of non-specific anxieties and concerns that are still present in your life.

You might find comfort in a fun and absorbing hobby (such as knit-ting or starting a new creative craft), or in a relaxing activity (like listening to soothing music or starting a good book.) Perhaps meditation or yoga or taking bubble baths is the way for you. Hugging a loved one or special pet can be very comforting as well.

Framing your self-talk in ways that are positive can be very comforting as well. For instance, you might make a list of things at which you excel. Or write kind thoughts directed at you on post-its and leave them around your living area. Or start a daily gratitude journal, acknowledging something for which you are grateful, each day.

These are just a few ways to self-soothe that have worked for me and some of my clients. (I have provided a partial list in the "Non-Food Ways to Self-Soothe" section in Part Four of this book.) The methods that people use to self-soothe are as unique as the reasons that drive them to seek such comfort. While some of these might work for you—and I encourage you to adopt the ones that do—there are probably several non-food-related comforts you can think of that particularly suit you.

Activity: Make a List of Non-Food Things That Comfort and Soothe You

Make a list of at least a dozen non-food ways you can create comfort to address and neutralize your emotion-triggers. You may include as many of my suggestions as you like, and I encourage you to come up with your own ideas.

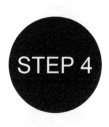

EMBRACING NEW COMFORT STRATEGIES

It is time to put what you have learned about your emotion triggers and the things that you find comforting, to work. As you feel these triggers being activated, guide your attention to the list of self-soothing strategies.

Activity: Record Your Emotion Triggers and Self-Soothing Response Actions

Create a Mood/Soothe Diary in your notebook, or download the Mood/Soothe Diary workbook pages from the Food Cuddler document in this book's online resource pages. (See sample diary fragment below.)

	When	Self-Soothing Response Actions
Example		

Think of this as a Mood/Food Diary without the "Food" part. The purpose of this diary is to keep a log of when you feel triggered by your emotions, and note all of your self-soothing (non-food) response actions to feeling triggered. If you find that you made the choice to comfort eat even though you wished you hadn't, just let any feelings of disappointment at your actions go; there is always the opportunity to make strong choices next time.

Remember, healing is a process. And learning to make helpful, healthy choices is a process as well. After all, and it bears repeating: my number one rule is, "Be kind to yourself."

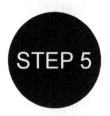

AFFIRM WHO YOU ARE

Finally, as you shift your self-soothing strategy away from primarily using comfort food to using other non-food methods to alleviate anxious feelings, celebrate and take ownership of your new mindful approach. In your notebook or workbook, write down the following statement, putting your name in the provided blank space.:

> I am_____. My heart is open and my attitude is flexible. Each day I remember that I love myself as I enjoy positive self-care activities that bring me comfort and enhance my life.

You may find it helpful to repeat this affirmation at those times when you feel an impulse to eat due to emotion triggers. Remember to read it to yourself each morning for at least a full month (though making it a habit for many more months is certainly recommended!)

7

THE FOOD WHISPERER

Some people, when emotionally upset, bring up the subject of whatever the issue happens to be for discussion...in a calm and rational manner. Other folks engage in loud, vocal conflict. And still others communicate their feelings of unhappiness either through stress eating, or through drastically restricting their intake of food.

THE FOOD WHISPERER

I can remember those not-so-long-ago days when big hair on women and girls was THE thing to have, at least for some people. Amy—a high school sophomore at the time—was one of those people. But then, one bright autumn Saturday, Amy's mom took the liberty of making an appointment at the hairdresser's for Amy. The mom, it seems, had decided that the big hair look was not for her Amy. And though Amy tried to convey her own preferences, she was no match for her very domineering mother. So by the end of the day, Amy's big hair had been cut short, her long, teased hair brusquely traded for an already out-of-style Dorothy Hamill wedge cut.

Amy did not kick up too much of a fuss; she did not want to disappoint her mom by contradicting her. So instead, she came home, took a seat at the kitchen table, and—though she was not hungry—she ate.

She ate as a way to disagree with her mom. She ate as a way to say, "I control my body."

She ate as a way to express feelings for which she had no words, and even if she did have the words, she didn't feel that she had the power in her family to speak them.

Years later, even as a grown woman, Amy admits that when she feels the need to impose some limits on her mother, to establish the healthy boundaries a grown child should be able to set around her parents, she reaches for the snack cupboard.

Amy's story is an all-too common one; I've heard different versions of it throughout my counseling career.

I've also counseled clients who have similar stories of struggles with parents or authority figures, but in these instances they do not communicate their feelings of upset and frustration through over-consuming food; they take their stands by *restricting* their food intake. Whether it's through over-consuming or restricting food consumption, many people who feel they have little or no control over important aspects of their lives will employ their use of food as the one facet of their existence they actually can control. For them, food comes as a way to demonstrate personal power, a method of silent protest that ends up being self-destructive, because those who use eating as a way to communicate often end up feeling powerless over food.

I helped Amy come up with words to protect her boundaries. She felt intimidated by her parents, and was afraid by asserting herself she was somehow disrespecting them. I pointed out that ideally, it's best to make all of our communications—especially those where we stand up for ourselves—with respect.

We discussed the importance of taking a moment to access our feelings when we feel an emotional challenge coming on. What is the feeling, and what is causing it? Then we talked about ways to address it. In this case, if negative emotions from an issue with another person come up, there is a powerful, simple tool to use: the "I" statement, which is a good way to neutrally stand up for your needs without making the other person wrong. You describe and take responsibility for your feelings, and explain their causes.

For example, Amy might have told her mom, "I feel frustrated when my preferences are ignored." There is no guarantee, of course, that her parents would be able to really hear and understand what she said, but the simple act of speaking her mind and using her voice could have helped Amy regain a sense of personal power and helped alleviate her sense of not being heard.

And whether or not her words were ignored, it was important to develop ways to soothe upset feelings other than eating for comfort.

(For Amy it was a warm bath.)

Self-Correction Toolkit for the Food Whisperer

To gain the greatest benefit from this toolkit, I highly recommend you obtain a dedicated notebook to do your work in, or download our toolkit worksheets by visiting www.whydidijusteatthat.com/resources and click on the "Food Whisperer" link for printable copies.

It is not unusual for people to use their behavior with food as a way to claim some sort of agency over their lives. Sometimes small children who bristle under controlling parents will restrict or over-indulge their intake of food as a way to claim some sort of power in the parent-child dynamic. It is interesting to note that whether one is over-consuming food or restricting intake, the underlying power-struggle dynamics are similar.

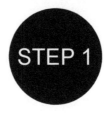

ADMIT...THEN COMMIT

Even as adults, many people use food as a way of pushing down their feelings. This is especially true when they feel that they don't have a voice. In time, food becomes a go-to mode of communicating frustration or anger, even when the person does not realize that that is what they're doing.

Write a Starting-Point Affirmation

Admit that you understand, for your highest good, that there needs to be a change in your style of thinking. Take some quiet time to acknowledge this, then record your thoughts in your notebook or the downloaded workbook pages. You might write down, "I am creating a healthy relationship with food as I open my heart up to clear and firm communication with the people in my world," to record your affirmation, then sign and date it. I also recommend finding a moment to look in the mirror and tell yourself this intention, explaining why—in your own words—this is important to you.

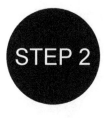

STEP 2

OBSERVE

Some people have learned earlier in life—incorrectly—that their opinions don't matter. Over time, they have become used to not sharing their preferences with others. In fact, they may feel they don't have a preference for much of anything, because they long ago stopped expressing preferences.

When we are small, our caregivers, teachers, and other mentors have a great deal of say over what we do and what we are able to do, and so their opinions are of critical importance to us. But as we grow up and mature, what our childhood authority figures think and say matters—in a practical sense—less and less. They no longer have direct control over our actions, yet we often give their opinions and thoughts much weight as if they did. We may refrain from pushing back against their opinions out of a wish to not offend them. We may take on their thoughts and opinions as our own without really examining them for accuracy or relevance. We may be so used to following their suggestions that we continue to do so through sheer habit.

When people have grown used to not being heard, they may be so accustomed to being ignored that it can be difficult for them to identify any of the times they feel ignored now. So the first thing I recommend is to make a list of all the instances, big and small, in which you have felt unheard. It is possible that (at first) only a couple of such instances will come to mind—or maybe none at all. For that reason, I recommend you take your time, and let these occasions pop into your memory as you open up your mind to recall them.

Activity: List Instances When You Feel/Felt Unheard

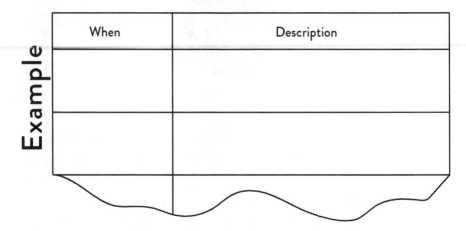

	When	Description
Example		

Additionally, note any instance during the next few days when what you say goes unacknowledged. Be aware of the dynamics in these situations; it is important to simply become familiar with the dynamics of these interactions. Pay particular attention to the times you wished you had found your voice but hadn't. Become aware, also, of what went on inside of you when you felt ignored, unacknowledged, or invalidated, when you felt there were strains of guilt or coercion in how they communicated their ideas, and felt discouraged from stating what was true for you.

Most importantly, make note of any or all times when you found yourself eating or restricting out of feelings of frustration or feelings of lack of control over your world.

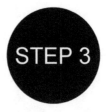

STEP 3

REWORK AND REFRAME

People who are uncomfortable speaking up for themselves may at first feel somewhat awkward in bringing the subject up in conversation. This is quite understandable, and while to speak up for ourselves often takes us out of our usual comfort zones, we can take our time flexing these new muscles.

Activity: Learning to be Heard

Go over the list you put together in Step Two, and identify times you felt unheard or disregarded, and identify the other person involved in that event. If appropriate and possible, approach them to communicate your feelings. Avoid "you" statements (as in, "You never listen to me, like last night at dinner when I said…") which is more likely to trigger a defensive reaction because the other person might take it as an attack. It is much more effective to use "I" statements (as in, "Last night at dinner, I felt unlistened to when I said…")

In the latter scenario, your statement may still trigger a defensive response, but it is more clear that you are describing how you feel, and are bringing up the subject for you and the other person to discuss and resolve together. (It is also possible that there was an occasion when you might have wanted to communicate something, but in the moment you could not find the words. You can still use this exercise to create the opportunity to state what you didn't say earlier).

Before you speak to the other person, it is a good idea to write out what you plan on saying. You need not have these notes with you when you do speak, but it is a good idea to have worked out in advance how you plan to broach the subject.

Of course, it might be that it is not appropriate and/or possible to address the issue with the other person. The other person may be, for example, a police officer who pulled you over the other day. Or the other person may be someone you have lost touch with, or is deceased, or is out of your life for another reason. And even though some of these people may no longer be physically in your life, their thoughts and opinions (or, at least our impression of these things) may live on as echoes in your mind. In any of these cases where the other person is unavailable, you might write out what you imagine what that dialogue between you two might look like.

Even though you cannot actually interact with them, going through the steps of communicating with them anyway can be very healing...even if no one else reads what you have written.

When you have a discussion with another person communicating these thoughts, you may or may not reach the results you hope for. While it is unfortunate to not achieve your goal every time, the most important aspect of this exercise is to become used to asserting your own needs and opinions to others in your life.

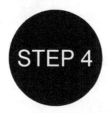

STEP 4

CHALLENGING OLD BEHAVIORS, UNHELPFUL INNER VOICES, ETC.

By now, you are probably aware of two related things: the times you have felt unheard, and your self-soothe responses to these feelings.

Ideally, after the previous exercises, you have begun to develop the wherewithal to be more self-assertive with your communications, either in the moment as the issue arises or discussing with growing confidence (and using "I" statements) after the fact. So, the Step Four activity is to go forward putting into action all that you've discovered in this chapter. Commit to using your voice in a matter-of-fact manner (with kindness and respect, if the situation calls for it). It will likely be hard at first...in fact, many get a stomachache while learning and practicing this challenging skill, but in time it does get easier.

To begin to assert your voice, find areas that are not contentious and simply ask for what you need. For example, ask someone to help clear the table or assist with the dishes. The more we practice asking for what we need, the easier it gets.

Those of us who had less of a voice growing up will undoubtedly find this more difficult. For some of us, it might even feel disrespectful or selfish. But the truth is, expressing our needs in a clear and unapologetic manner is a form of self-care. The more we're able to ask for what we need, the more self-empowered we will feel. We will not always get what we ask for, but to simply ask is a pathway to feeling more fulfilled and having a stronger sense of self—and a way toward not needing food as a way of expressing unfulfilled needs.

A final word to the Food Whisperer: Of course, I understand that trying to secure comfort either through eating (when you are not hungry) or restricting food (when your body does need to eat) is a difficult habit to break. So, I recommend everyone think of non-food-related ways to self-soothe. Many people find creative endeavors or indulging in comforting self-care regimens to be extremely soothing. There is a list at the back of the book with some ideas. It is a good idea to have a few self-soothe ideas in the back of your mind for you to pull out when you feel triggered for any reason, especially those discussed in this chapter.

NUTRITION BYTE: Everyone has a right to speak, have an opinion, and express wants and needs. Some people whose inner voice drives them to feel insecure may have a harder time speaking up for themselves; awareness of this dynamic is the first step toward healing!

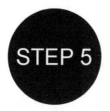

STEP 5

AFFIRM WHO YOU ARE

Being able to communicate your needs after a long period of not being able to do so is super-challenging. Even as you find your voice, there may be days when you feel your voice shut down. This is part of the process, and the trick is to forgive yourself for not being perfect and "get back onto the horse."

Obviously, a big part of transitioning to more confident communication levels stems from your mindset. We opened this section with an affirmation of intent, and now we'll close this chapter with an affirmation of acknowledgement and centering.

In your notebook or "Food Whisperer" workbook pages, write down the following statement, putting your name in the provided blank space. Repeat it to yourself every day in quiet moments, perhaps as you lie in bed in the morning or at the end of your day, or while meditating or exercising. Try to do this every day for at least a month. If you forget, that's fine, just forgive yourself and pick up where you left off.

I am_____. My heart is open, I have a healthy relationship with food, and I am worthy enough to share my thoughts, needs and desires with clarity; I am heard.

Even if you feel uncomfortable or don't fully believe this statement at first, remember that in order to grow, we must become clear on what we aspire to be.

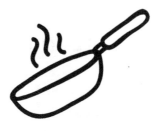

8

THE GET-IT-WHILE-YOU-CAN EATER

I was once told about the time some friends took their mentor out to dinner. He didn't eat a lot, and as the plates were being cleared away, his friends asked him if he had had enough to eat.

"Nah," he said, "I think I'll eat again tomorrow."

Not everyone has such a straightforward attitude when it comes to food and portions. For some, feelings of scarcity and lack distort mealtime eating strategies. Food, after all, is a complex part of our lives. Its role for each of us as individuals extends far beyond food's simple function as fuel. For example, while an adequate amount of food is necessary to maintain our health, for many people the given amount of food also reflects a gut-level basic sense of abundance and security. People who grew up with feelings of scarcity may find that feelings of never having enough to eat persist years after the causes of these feelings have ceased to be an issue. And for people with a tendency to have emotions triggered by anxieties of lack, food is often a go-to source of comfort.

THE GET-IT-WHILE-YOU-CAN EATER

Chris was a 63-year-old male who came to my office looking for a way to lose weight, which—at the time of his initial visit—had crept up to a number he felt ashamed of. Chris reported that he had decided that, once and for all, it was time he get serious about changing his lifestyle. His job as a general contractor required him to spend a great deal of time in his car, driving from worksite to worksite. As such, his on-the-go meals and snacks were pretty haphazard; stopping wherever he could grab a quick bite at whatever eating establishment happened to be on his route. His large stature—a tad under six feet, seven inches—put a lot of pressure on his feet, which made it increasingly difficult for him to do a whole lot of walking.

We began by discussing how food was handled in his upbringing. As the oldest of 10 children in a modest income home, the kids' mealtime motto was, "If you snooze, you lose!" When your baby brother gets more food than you do as a growing adolescent, Chris learned, you learn to get into the food line early and value every bite. This set up a dynamic that had Chris regularly rushing to always be first at the table come mealtime.

When he grew up and was on his own, Chris maintained his childhood habit of making sure to eat something before feeling hunger, just in case he got hungry later on and there was no food available.

Chris also mentioned something that was not directly food-related, but seemed to me as relevant to his state of mind when it came to "getting his share." When he was in middle school, his whole family was planning on going on a week-long summer's vacation in the mountains. Unfortunately, Chris broke his arm riding his bike just after school let out; his parents decided to have his grandmother babysit him at home while the rest of his family—parents and siblings—went on the scheduled vacation without him. Chris admitted that to this day he gets a little knot in his stomach when he feels like he is getting left out. This ingrained feeling of "lack" helped him achieve a certain amount of professional success, but it did leave him with certain less-than-helpful habits, notably when it came to food and eating.

An important tool in assisting clients is helping them gain awareness of their actions and maybe some insights into the choices they make. As we teased apart and processed what was driving Chris's eating behavior, he was able to take time to approach meals and snacks differently. He was able to make time to pack lunches and snacks to take with him when he visited his company's work sites.

He would work regular supermarket stops into his weekly routine to make sure he had healthful and satisfying foods available, making it easier to prepare his meals and snacks. He began to focus on experiencing his own internal cues of hunger and fullness, learning to eat intuitively instead of relying on the clock or reacting from old childhood fears of lack to determine when he ate. Though I did not put him on a deprivation diet to lose weight, the healthier behaviors he adopted made him feel more fit. In time, he reported to me with some measure of pride that one of his greatest accomplishments was when he realized he was able to do a 45-minute walk as a leisurely exercise and his feet didn't bother him.

Self-Correction Toolkit for the Get-It-While-You-Can Eater

To gain the greatest benefit from this toolkit, I highly recommend you obtain a dedicated notebook to do your work in, or download our toolkit worksheets by visiting www.whydidijusteatthat.com/resources and click on the "Get-It-While-You-Can Eater" link for printable copies.

For those with a history of food insecurity, the effects of past memories of deprivation can run very deep...even if food insecurity is no longer a problem today. It makes perfect sense that people who struggled with feelings of lack in their formative years might continue to obey the impulse to eat more than is actually required by their current circumstances.

On some deep level, they have been conditioned to expect that food may be scarce in the near future. Such unquestioned conditioning tends to endure, and the longer this state of mind endures, the more challenging it is to break. This is one of the more difficult behaviors to break because the memories and traumas run so deep.

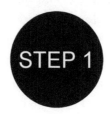

ADMIT...THEN COMMIT

Write a Starting-Point Affirmation

Admit that you understand, for your highest good, that there needs to be a change in your relationship with food. Take some quiet time to acknowledge this then record your thoughts in your notebook or the downloaded workbook pages. You might write down, "I am open to feelings of abundance and listening to my body's nutrition-related wisdom," in the space marked Affirmations below, then sign and date it. I also recommend finding a moment to look in the mirror and tell yourself of this intention. Also make a note explaining why—in your own words—that this is important to you on the space allotted below the affirmation.

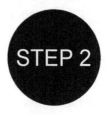

OBSERVE

When facing an eating issue—any eating issue, really—the first step is to pay closer attention to your habits, in writing, over a period of at least a week. Becoming aware of the dynamics of an issue is a major first step toward resolving that issue.

Activity: Write a Letter to Yourself as the Child You Once Were

This observation step comes in two parts: for the first part, in your notebook or the downloaded workbook pages, write a letter to yourself from the point of view of you as a child. Describe what mealtime felt like. Was there a sense of lack? Were there siblings to compete with over a limited amount of food? Explore what it felt like to not know if you were going to have enough to eat.

Activity: Mood/Food Diary

The second part of the observation step is using a really useful tool called a Mood/Food Diary. On these pages of your diary, keep track of what you eat, when you eat, and your levels of hunger and fullness for each meal or snack.

It is important that before you start your diary, you first understand how to track levels of hunger and fullness. I recommend creating a hunger/fullness meter, a scale that measures the range of sensations from feeling hungry to feeling full in increments of 1 to 10, with "1" being super hungry and "10" feeling excessively, uncomfortably full.

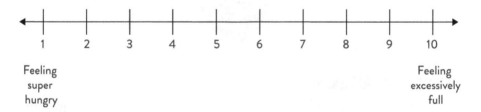

| 1 | 2 | 3 | 4 | 5 | 6 | 7 | 8 | 9 | 10 |

Feeling super hungry   Feeling excessively full

Download the Mood/Food Diary workbook pages from the "Get it While You Can Eater" document in this book's online resource pages. Or, to create a Mood/Food Diary in your notebook, use the sample diary fragment below as a guide.)

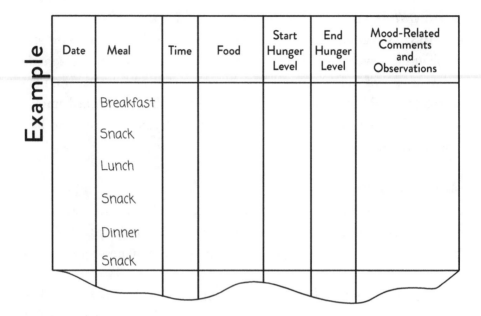

	Date	Meal	Time	Food	Start Hunger Level	End Hunger Level	Mood-Related Comments and Observations
Example		Breakfast					
		Snack					
		Lunch					
		Snack					
		Dinner					
		Snack					

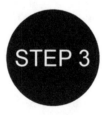

STEP 3

REWORK AND REFRAME

After you have completed the letter from the "childhood you" to yourself today, and filled out the diary, the next step takes you forward.

Activity: Write a Letter to Your Child Self

In your notebook or the downloaded workbook pages, write a letter from your adult self to your child self. Be compassionate and understanding of the feelings of the past you, with compassion and understanding as seen from your current perspective of safety and security. Comfort that "past you" with the reassuring knowledge that scarcity and lack are no longer the case in your life. Include in your letter any observations you were able to draw from your Mood/Food Diary about old patterns that may no longer serve you.

Explore what it now feels like to be confident that you now *do* have enough to eat. And most of all, communicate with that precious child who is the past you that they are safe.

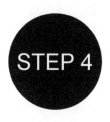

STEP 4

CHALLENGING OLD BEHAVIORS, UNHELPFUL INNER VOICES, ETC.

It is important that both you and your body begin to trust that you will be fed when you need food. Spend a couple of weeks following the Eating Abundance Schedule laid out below, keeping in mind these important points:

1. Have something to eat every two and a half to three and a half hours.
2. Remember to honor your feelings of hunger and fullness.
3. Take care to eat slowly, because it takes some time for your digestive system to relay the information to your brain that your stomach is full.
4. When you are no longer hungry, take a moment to tell yourself something like "I'm at a '7' on the hunger/fullness scale and I choose to stop eating, because I can always have more later when I feel hungry."

(You can fill in the proper details of time and dates as suits your own specific schedule.)

Download the Food Diary workbook pages from the "Get-It-While-You-Can Eater" document in this book's online resource pages. Or, to create a Food Diary in your notebook, use the sample diary fragment below as a guide: your diary should have separate columns, listing Date, Meal,

Time, Food Consumed, and a Reminder to Tell Yourself at Each Meal. That last column should contain an affirmation: "I choose to stop eating when I am no longer hungry, because I know I can eat more later when I do feel hungry."

	Date	Meal	Time	Food Consumed	Remember to tell yourself at each meal:
Example		Breakfast Snack Lunch Snack Dinner Snack			I choose to stop eating when I am no longer hungry, because I know I can have more later when I do feel hungry.

Our relationship with food is an echo of the most important relationship in our lives: namely, our relationship with ourselves. That critical relationship is determined by our understanding of who we are, and that understanding in turn is determined by the stories we tell ourselves about ourselves.

People who formed their sense of self—and how it relates to the world— in a context of lack and scarcity may have that sense of lack permeating many of their self-identifying stories. That learned sense of lack (even if no longer accurate) can govern many of their choices, including eating habits. In cases like the "Get-It-While-You-Can Eater," it is usually important, then, to rewrite the self-identifying stories by evolving a few key beliefs.

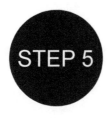

AFFIRM WHO YOU ARE

In order to progress, it is often important that we change our limiting beliefs to something more expansive. We will end this chapter with a tool that can help you rewrite part of your self-understanding: an affirmation for you to repeat to yourself every day for at least a month. In your notebook or workbook, write down the following statement, putting your name in the provided blank space.:

> I am _____. I trust that my body's intuitive wisdom knows what is best for it. Today and every day I honor my hunger and fullness cues and take just enough food to satisfy my hunger, slowly enjoying it, secure in the knowledge that food is plentiful in my life and I have access to wholesome nourishment whenever I wish.

Sometimes as major personal shifts lie ahead, many of us feel resistance regarding things like affirmations. We may feel it is foolish, or that it won't work. My strong advice is that this last tool is a critical one in cementing in the change you have worked so hard to achieve.

> **NUTRITION BYTE:** If we choose not to surrender to old feelings of negativity, but instead acknowledge things—great and small—that spark appreciation, we can embrace a wider experience of gratitude; fully living in gratitude is about choosing the context that colors our world. We are the stories we tell ourselves about ourselves.

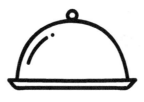

9

THE ONCE-A-DAY DINER

Some folks habitually eat little to no breakfast, little to no lunch; in fact—aside from coffee and a trip to the vending machine—little or no food at all. But when they get home from work feeling famished, they'll reach for everything in sight for the next few hours.

The mechanics of this make sense. Physiologically, the brains of people who restrict intake all day are functionally starving and cry out for food by day's end. When food is finally made available, bodies and brains crave as much as possible. The reaction to this mini-famine is to eat and eat, way past the point of satiation.

The problem with eating most of your food later in the day means that your body has not had an adequate source of nutrients for several hours. Metabolism slows when it perceives starvation, making it hard to stop eating once we've started. The net effect has us consuming more food than would otherwise have been eaten all day, craving in particular foods with fat content that could see us through future periods of "starvation."

Additionally, this habit of eating can aggravate such harmful conditions as acid reflux, because going to sleep soon after eating large amounts of food may make it more likely that stomach contents will push up into the esophagus and cause indigestion and burning.

THE ONCE-A-DAY DINER

Harriet, a 64-year-old married woman, came to my office for help. She was unhappy with her weight, her body, and the way she felt about it. As we spoke, it soon became clear that her problems with her body were only part of everything that felt wrong in her world. She shared with me that her home life was boring and joyless and that she felt separation from her husband was imminent. Her workday wasn't exactly boring, but it was stressful and disheartening: two of her colleagues were out on maternity leave, and Harriet was stretched extremely thin trying to keep up with both of their workloads as well as staying on top of her own. Is it any wonder she spent her days feeling beaten up by life and unnourished?

"It's easy," I pointed out, "to get overwhelmed in the barrage of challenging details. Can we step through a typical day looking at specifics?"

We began to review her daily routine, and I asked my usual opening nutrition-related question: "What's the first time in the day that you usually eat?"

Her answer was that her first actual meal was around 3:00 p.m.— if you could call it a meal. She would have several cups of coffee with sugar throughout the morning and by the time mid-afternoon would roll around, she'd be famished. So around 3:00 p.m. she would hit the vending machines, eat leftover muffins or bagels from the office kitchen, basically snacking on "anything she could find" until going home at 6:00 p.m., where she would continue to graze in front of the TV until she went to bed around 11:00 p.m.

It was as though she was having a single meal a day, lasting eight hours and consisting of countless tiny courses, some of which had low fiber and little nutritional density. This pattern was a familiar (though exaggerated) version of a pattern I often see in my office: food restriction, followed by binge eating. She explained that she had always grazed and, from where I sat, it seemed she didn't really know how to eat structured meals. She had no nutrition strategy, and she was so frustrated and unhappy with her life that she had lost the wherewithal to pursue better coping skills.

I helped Harriet come up with a few acceptable options for a smaller first meal, since she had never been much of a breakfast eater. She chose 8:00 a.m. as a goal mealtime. I suggested she put a rubber band on her left wrist at 8:00 a.m., signaling the beginning of mealtime, and that she move it to her right hand by 8:30 a.m., after she had finished eating, signaling that her meal was over. Using alarms on her smartphone I asked her to repeat this at 10:30 a.m. (some nuts for snack), 1:00 p.m. (lunch), 4:00 p.m. (snack), and 7:00 p.m. (dinner).

The combination of the visual cue (the rubber band,) the audible alarm reminder, and the structuring of her mealtimes taught her how to nourish her body throughout the day, dramatically decreasing her impulse to graze all night.

Self-Correction Toolkit for the Once-a-Day Diner

> To gain the greatest benefit from this toolkit, I highly recommend you obtain a dedicated notebook to do your work in, or download our toolkit worksheets by visiting www.whydidijusteatthat.com/resources and click on the "Once-a-Day-Diner" link for printable copies.

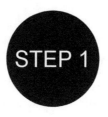

ADMIT...THEN COMMIT

As is the case for so many eaters, sticking to preparation and planning is key to moving forward to healing this issue.

Write a Starting-Point Affirmation

Admit that you understand, for your highest good, that there needs to be a change in your style of thinking. Take some quiet time to acknowledge this, then record your thoughts in your notebook or the downloaded workbook pages. You might write down, "I am becoming more aware of what my body needs, and embracing gentle structure throughout my day to best serve my life and eating habits," in the space marked Affirmations below, then sign and date it. I also recommend finding a moment to look in the mirror and tell yourself of this intention, and why—in your own words—that this is important to you.

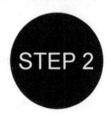

OBSERVE

After committing to change, the next step revolves around taking stock of where you are. (After all, you cannot move from where you are not.) So let's take some time creating a snapshot awareness of what is going on in your life related to your current relationship with the daily practice of eating, using two worksheets.

Exercise #1: In your notebook or downloaded workbook pages, take stock of how your eating habits have shifted over the years. In our younger years, our meals and snacks are generally established by parents or caregivers. Over time, some people maintain some sort of regular feeding schedule while others let their eating routines dissipate. Try to figure out why you shifted into your current eating pattern using the following three questions as prompts.

1. When you last had a conventional three-meal-a-day eating schedule, (with or without snacks,) how was your life structured?
2. What is your eating schedule now?

3. What aspects of your current life promote your typical eating schedule, or lack of a schedule?

Exercise #2: Download the Food Schedule Diary workbook pages from the "Once-a-Day Diner" document in this book's online resource pages. Or, to create a Food Schedule Diary in your notebook, use the sample diary fragment below as a guide.)

Keep your food schedule diary for one week. Track what you eat, how much, and at what times. This is not a calorie-counting exercise; its purpose is to get a clear picture of how you eat and your typical intake of nutrition.

Day 1

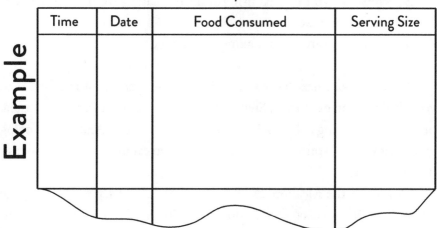

Time	Date	Food Consumed	Serving Size

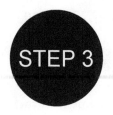

REWORK AND REFRAME

After a week, go back and read your three answers you wrote on the first worksheet. In your notebook or downloaded workbook pages, answer the three follow-up questions below:

1. What has changed in your life that changed your approach to eating?
2. How can you re-establish a healthier eating routine? What steps might you take?
3. Will you commit to making the change?

The final worksheet has you creating another version of the food diary you filled in as an exercise in Step 2, with a few notable differences. Instead of each section being a day, each section is an entire week. And instead of logging what you eat, you are going to plan what you eat in advance, following a defined schedule.

Download the Meal/Snacks Planned Schedule Diary workbook pages from the "Once-a-Day Diner" document in this book's online resource pages. Or, to create a Meal/Snacks Planned Schedule Diary in your notebook, use the sample diary fragment on the following page as a guide. Instead of creating a diary covering seven days, this exercise will have you covering seven weeks.

Day 1

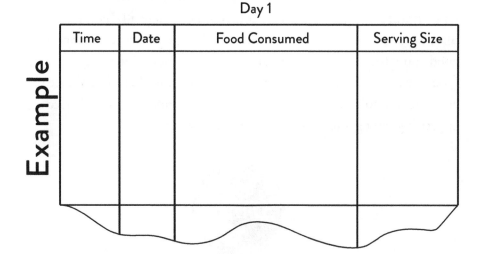

Time	Date	Food Consumed	Serving Size

I realize that after being in an unstructured habit of eating for an extended period of time, abruptly imposing a strict eating schedule on you—and then expecting you to follow—it would probably be unrealistic and set you up for failure. With that in mind, I recommend we slowly fill the schedule in, over a period of weeks. Each week can see new additions added to the schedule. By the end of the process you'll have adopted a plan that you've grown comfortable with, and at your own pace.

For example: For **Week 1** you might eat as you normally do, but additionally schedule nutritious snacks for the morning and afternoon time slots (snacks consisting of things like nuts, seeds, or dried fruit.)

Then for **Week 2** you might add to this schedule a lunch slot around midday (things like a grilled chicken sandwich with lettuce, tomato and avocado, or a chef's salad) and also a limited late snack a couple of hours or so before you go to bed (something like hummus and carrot pieces, or sliced banana and a spoonful of almond butter.)

On **Week 3**, add a breakfast slot (somewhere between the time you wake up and 9:30am.) An example of breakfast foods might be a bowl of oatmeal with a dollop of nut butter for protein, or perhaps an egg or two on whole grain toast and a sliced apple.

...and so on, adding meals or snacks until all the time slots on your schedules are filled, and you are ready to follow them all. (No need to put undue pressure on yourself to follow the schedule *perfectly*; good enough is good enough). Of course, you are not locking yourself into any particular foods, just committing to eating in specific time slots. In fact, embrace variety in food choices; as long as the choices are more or less balanced and appetizing, you get to choose whatever you want!

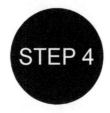

STEP 4

MOVING FORWARD

One of the key aspects to maintaining positive eating strategies is adequate and well-considered preparation. So it is important to regularly do some advance meal and snack planning twice a week. Pick two days a week to plan your meals and snacks and stick to it.

Planning is the first step, procuring all the ingredients for your planned menu is the next. Set up one major food shop a week, and then a smaller one to fill in additional perishables three or four days later. The more planning you do in advance, the easier it is to operate your eating strategy. For example, buy or prepare six grilled chicken breasts. Wrap each one individually and place them in the freezer. Then you'll have something to defrost to go in a sandwich, dice into a salad, shred inside a taco. More importantly, if an adequate variety of food is not regularly available to grab or use, it will be too easy to slip into old, adverse habits.

One last note: Since most *Once-a-Day Diners* have become accustomed to eating at night, it's important to plan some night-time fun activities to take the place of the eating (playing games online, starting a craft, or reading.) Snacking while watching TV is a pretty common habit and is important to avoid as it promotes mindless eating.

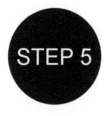

AFFIRM WHO YOU ARE

We began these exercises with a statement of acknowledgment, and we'll end with an affirmation—lock in your new eating strategy by celebrating and making this statement your own.

In your notebook or workbook, write down the following statement, putting your name in the provided blank space:

> I am_____. My heart is open, and my attitude is flexible. I am gratefully putting into practice the planning, organizing, and action steps embracing healthy nutrition habits for my highest good.

It can be very effective to repeat your affirmation to yourself each morning for at least a full month (though making it a habit for many more months is certainly recommended.)

Make it part of your daily schedule!

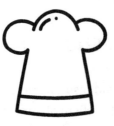

10

THE PENDULUM EATER

This type of eater is all too common.

Ideally, a healthy eating approach recognizes the value of consistency. Unfortunately, some types of eaters are always looking for the next great diet; the next guaranteed way to shed pounds quickly. They'll swing from restrictive diet plan to restrictive diet plan, perhaps finding themselves losing weight, only to regain that weight and more. Other eaters see-saw back and forth between harsh restriction and binge eating, then it's back to restrictive eating once again. What all these eaters have in common is a scattershot relationship with food.

The problem with this, of course, is that our bodies really do best when we eat in a predictable and consistent sort of way. When our eating habits are consistent, our body can trust that it will get fed, regularly, with a proper variety and blend of nutrients.

THE PENDULUM EATER

Michael was a 62-year-old insurance agent who reluctantly came to see me upon the urging of another client of mine. After gaining over 100 pounds while "dieting," Michael had just about decided to throw in the towel and give up. He was beyond frustrated and confessed to me that he desperately wanted to live in a smaller body. At our first session, I questioned him about his eating habits and he described an all-too-common scenario: "I grab a cup of coffee at Starbucks in the morning, then find something light, like maybe a deli sandwich for my lunch. Dinner time, I try to be *good*...but once I start to eat, it's like I can't stop. I'll eat dinner, and then snack on this and that, basically until I'm in bed. Sometimes I'm not even really paying attention to what I'm eating until it's all finished. Anyway, so then I get to bed, all upset at myself once again."

The first thing we did was discuss the restrict-binge phenomenon, that pendulum-swinging dynamic wherein someone eats very little for a period of time, followed by an episode (or more than one episode) of larger-scale consumption. While sometimes the restricting is due to some sort of deprivation dieting, restriction can also be rooted in poor planning and ignoring of hunger cues. Regardless of the cause, the feeling of deprivation tends to trigger an urge to take in a lot of food to make up for what the body misinterprets as potential famine. Whether the eating habits are well-planned or poorly disciplined, our bodies always try their best to get consistent nourishment and will prompt our impulse to eat accordingly.

I explained how our bodies are wired for consistency and predictability with food. I explained how restriction, being excessively hungry will almost always trigger an overeating response. Together, we designed a consistent nutrition intake plan for Michael that included three daily meals plus one or two snacks. I also assigned him techniques with which he could learn to eat intuitively.

By eating intuitively he eventually became aware of his body's hunger and fullness cues, and this awareness helped him eat based on his body's needs and not based on emotions or old behavioral triggers. For example, we gave numerical rankings to his relative levels of hunger and fullness; that is, "level 1" is so hungry the hunger pangs are uncomfortable and "level 10" is so full as to be loosen-the-belt-a-notch uncomfortable. I recommended that he not let his hunger level drop below "level 3" before eating and stop eating around a "level 7."

Additionally, I had him keep a food diary of his meals and snacks, maintaining a hunger-fullness level score at the beginning, middle, and end of each eating experience. He also made note of his moods at each meal or snack. Writing out what he was eating alongside how he was feeling helped him observe the connection between his thoughts and his eating impulses, and helped encourage him to stay present and in the moment.

Self-Correction Toolkit for the Pendulum Eater

> To gain the greatest benefit from this toolkit, I highly recommend you obtain a dedicated notebook to do your work in, or download our toolkit worksheets by visiting www.whydidijusteatthat.com/resources and click on the "Pendulum Eater" link for printable copies.

First, a little background. We know that intake restriction has a negative physiological effect on our brain. It signals famine, which causes our metabolism to decrease in an attempt to conserve whatever energy we can in an environment of diminishing nutrition expectations. When the pendulum swings back to more available food, our physiology urges us to eat more because our brain is wired for survival and wants us to make up for what we missed. Much of what we eat is stored as body fat in anticipation of the next famine.

Our bodies cannot tell the difference between a real, life-threatening famine, and a self-imposed restrictive diet. When we restrict and lose weight we lose fat and muscle, but when we put the weight back on we gain back only fat. Over a period of time our percentage of lean body mass goes down while our percentage of fat goes up. This higher fat percentage means a slower metabolic rate, because muscle needs more calories to maintain itself than fat does. This is how pendulum eating actually decreases the amount of muscle we had in the first place, lowering our metabolism.

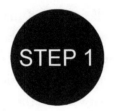

ADMIT...THEN COMMIT

The effects of being a Pendulum Eater are often years in the making and will take time to reverse. But we can move away from where we are, and getting off that swinging pendulum is a good idea at any time. So, how do we get away from pendulum eating? Let's start small.

Write a Starting-Point Affirmation

First, start by acknowledging that up until now, you have been a pendulum eater and that you understand that there needs to be a change in your relationship with food. Take some quiet time to acknowledge this, then record your thoughts in your notebook or the downloaded workbook pages. You might write down, "I am reclaiming a healthy, consistent manner of eating and relationship with food," in the space marked Affirmations below, then sign and date it. I also recommend finding a moment to look in the mirror and tell yourself of this intention, and why—in your own words—that this is important to you.

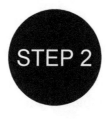

OBSERVE

The observation phase of addressing this issue comes in two parts: noting the past, and then tracking the present.

Worksheets

Exercise 1. Reflection often has the ability to put things in perspective, and through hindsight we might have a chance to learn about which of our choices worked, and which didn't. So make a list of the eating strategies—or "diets"—you've been on over the last five to 10 years. Include your best recollection of how long you were on each one, and then what happened when the diet ended. Did you switch to a new diet? Did you go off and then fall into a binge-eating cycle for a while? Reflect on the effectiveness of the diets. What can you take away from your personal diet history? Have any of your past diets gotten you to the place of meeting your long-term nutrition goals?

	Eating Strategy	Time Period	Comments
Example	Grapefruit Diet	3 weeks	Temporary weight loss
	Cabbage Soup Diet	4 days	Felt very bloated, hard to stay with

Exercise 2. After you've completed the worksheet, turn your attention to keeping a Food Diary and observe how you're eating from day to day. Download the Food Diary workbook pages from the "Pendulum Eater" document in this book's online resource pages, or, to create a Food Diary in your notebook, use the sample diary fragment below as a guide.

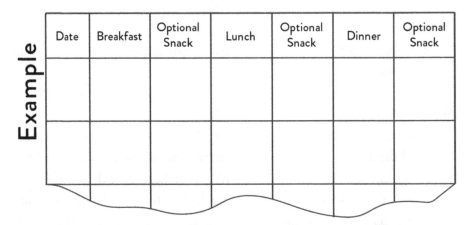

Example	Date	Breakfast	Optional Snack	Lunch	Optional Snack	Dinner	Optional Snack

After a week, consider what you have written in your diary. Is your intake fairly consistent? Is it fairly nourishing? Is it fairly satisfying? Do you have binge days, cheat days and days to be "good"? Do your habits feel truly satisfying, or overly-restrictive, or chaotic? Are you ready to get a handle on your relationship with food and eating?

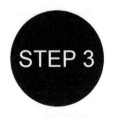

STEP 3

REWORK AND REFRAME

Most diets are based on deprivation, and deprivation often leads to binge eating. With that in mind, isn't it well past time to throw out the diet mentality? Sure, that's easier said than done, but studies have proven over and over again that diets don't work.[1] Very few people who go on a diet will actually keep their weight off in subsequent years. To put this in perspective, if I told you that the airplane you're about to board has a very poor chance of getting to its destination in one piece, would you really want to get on that plane?

I'd rather walk!

Keeping our travel metaphor for a while longer, you've probably heard that expression, "Every great journey starts with one small step." Well, this is true of internal journeys as well. I recommend you try to find a few small steps and changes that can be made over the long run to help you meet your nutrition goals.

So, how about if we replace the concept of dieting with something more effective? Let's borrow a term from the business world. In the early 1980s, the concept of "S.M.A.R.T. goals" appeared in business journals; S.M.A.R.T. being an acronym for Specific, Measurable, Attainable, Relevant, and Time-Bound[2]. This clear and exact way of framing a workable strategy is a great place to start small steps toward new relationships with food and with eating.

Worksheet

List three positive diet changes that you'd like to commit to, and position them as S.M.A.R.T. goals. For example, a smart goal might be "I will eat two meals of fish a week" or "I will eat three servings of vegetables a day, five days per week." You can see how this is much more concrete than simply saying, "I will eat more vegetables." (That approach would be non-S.M.A.R.T.: not specific, measurable, or time-bound.)

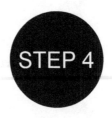

STEP 4

STEPPING AWAY FROM BEHAVIORS THAT NO LONGER SERVE US

Making a few small changes at a time can add up to produce long-term results. The key here is that they need to be ongoing.

The next worksheet is similar to your Food Diary, only this one will function as your Meal Planner. Download the Meal Planner workbook pages from the "Pendulum Eater" document in this book's online resource pages, or, to create a Meal Planner in your notebook, use the sample diary fragment below as a guide.

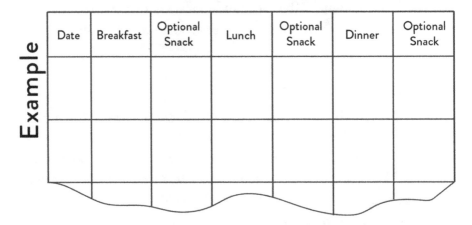

	Date	Breakfast	Optional Snack	Lunch	Optional Snack	Dinner	Optional Snack
Example							

Examine your S.M.A.R.T. list, and take the ideas listed to be included in your meal plan. Just include the three S.M.A.R.T. suggestions; don't make any more until you can work these into your eating habits. Small, achievable steps are the goal. You don't need to create a total, inflexible meal plan, but what you do include is, ideally, Specific, Measurable, Attainable, Relevant, and Time-Bound.

Steady and predictable eating habits soon give our bodies a consistent message that nourishing foods will be offered regularly. A good rule of thumb is to commit to a nourishing meal plan 80 percent of the time, which is to say one portion of some fun foods for every four portions of nutritious fare.

Finding a "forever way to eat" is the best way to get off the pendulum. It may take your body several months or even years to trust and know it's going to get fed consistently, so be patient. Most people don't end up with body dissatisfaction overnight. It builds and so it needs to slowly dissipate for long-term success.

A big part of that is reacquainting yourself with your internal hunger and fullness cues, learning to eat when hungry and stop eating when satisfied. As I mentioned earlier in this chapter—and elsewhere in this book—a major part of moving beyond the limitations caused by eating issues is to become aware of your hunger/fullness meter.

Your hunger/fullness meter is a scale that measures the range of sensations from feeling hungry to feeling full in increments of 1 to 10, with "1" being super hungry and "10" feeling excessively full.

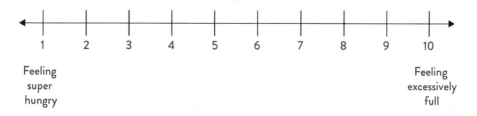

As you begin to pay close attention to what your body is experiencing regarding the spectrum spanning hunger and fullness, eating intuitively will help you regulate your intake in a way that helps you feel good about food physically, as well as emotionally.

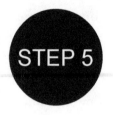

STEP 5

AFFIRM WHO YOU ARE

We began these exercises with a statement of acknowledgment, and we'll end with an affirmation for you to repeat to yourself every day for at least a month, especially if you find yourself feeling anxious over this uncomfortably (at first) new approach to your eating strategies. In your notebook or workbook, write down the following statement, putting your name in the provided blank space.:

> I am _____ . I trust in my body's growing wisdom in knowing what is best for it. I eat intuitively, embracing wholesome nourishment while enjoying a wide variety of foods that feed my body and soul.

Try to repeat your new affirmation to yourself every day in quiet moments, perhaps as you lie in bed in the morning or at the end of your day, or while meditating or exercising. Try to do this every day for at least a month. If you forget, that's fine, just forgive yourself and pick up where you left off. Even if you don't fully believe this statement at first, remember that in order to grow, we must become clear on what we aspire to be.

11

THE PRESSURE-COOKER EATER

We all experience stress from time to time, and each of us reacts to it in our own particular way. Stress has, at one time or other, affected the eating patterns of many—if not most—of us. But for some, managing stress is a huge, continuing challenge. It is difficult to overstate the role that food plays as a consequence of stress in the lives of many people. Some people find they lose their appetites when stressed or upset, while others crave sweets or carbs or fatty foods. Whether they eat too much or too little, for too many, stress is an ongoing problem that plays havoc with many aspects of their lives. When I think of "pressure-cooker eaters," I think of an actual pressure cooker. As we gently apply the release valve and let some steam out, we're able to calm down our system.

THE PRESSURE-COOKER EATER

Jerry, 45, was sent to me after dropping so much weight that his primary physician initially wondered if there was a medical cause. After running a few preliminary tests, it was determined that his rapid and sudden weight loss was likely due to loss of appetite that took hold on the heels of his contentious divorce.

Very often, if we don't take care of ourselves due to upset feelings, the fact that we don't feel like taking care of ourselves leads to more upset feelings. I helped Jerry set up a snacking schedule that worked for him, consisting of nuts, seeds, and dried fruit, foods that are nutritionally and calorically dense. We discussed the troubling weight loss stemming from his poor eating choices. He was able to understand that his self-sabotaging self-care was actually an expression of his anger at himself over the end of his marriage.

Jerry's case notwithstanding, much more common, of course, is for people to eat to excess while under stress. Beth, a graduate student, told me that when conflicting school deadlines loomed ominously, she practically relocated her bedroom into her refrigerator, for all the time she spent there.

Food often serves as a distraction, dissipating our focus. Sometimes when we are feeling strong emotions—whether it is related to stress, anxiety, even happiness—emotional energy builds up, demanding some sort of release. We feel the need to do something, anything. Getting food, preparing it, eating it...all these things take some level of thought and action, and can distract us from whatever it is that is stressing us. Also, certain foods may remind us of simpler, happy times, and the sense-memory we get from eating these foods (often, so-called "comfort foods") tend to have soothing properties.

Since we can control what we put—or don't put—into our mouths, in times when everything else appears to be out of control, eating can seem like one area that we do have some sort of control, and by taking that control some people may feel more in charge of at least one aspect of their lives. If we feel uncared for by the outer world, eating can feel like a demonstration of self-care. Stress eating is a blend of learned responses—if a parent stress-ate, it is more likely that you will— and inborn tendencies.

What do stress eating and nourishment have in common? Well, nothing!

Restricting food because you are too upset to eat obviously can lead to health problems. Conversely, it is ironic that stress eating often leaves one feeling more stressed after a bout of stress eating, especially if it is stress-binging, which may offer someone a little bit of comfort in the short run, but much more regret and despair in the long run. So in the end, it is not even effective at managing stress.

Self-Correction Toolkit for the Pressure-Cooker Eater

To gain the greatest benefit from this toolkit, I highly recommend you obtain a dedicated notebook to do your work in, or download our toolkit worksheets by visiting www.whydidijusteatthat.com/resources and click on the "Pressure-Cooker Eater" link for printable copies.

No matter how stress affects your eating—whether it causes you to overeat or undereat—the solution is to first acknowledge that the strong stress-related emotions that are being processed have nothing to do with the acquisition of nutrition; and of course, the acquisition of nutrition is the basic point of eating. Learning to separate the two—and finding other ways to manage the stress—is the first step to getting pressure-cooker eating under control.

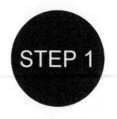

ADMIT...THEN COMMIT

The first step toward healing, of course, is to acknowledge that there is a problem, and recognizing that changes in behavior must be made. Since it is true that change in behavior cannot be made without first a proactive change in attitude, I always like to start people with owning where they are and holding a clear idea of where they wish to go.

Write a Starting-Point Affirmation

Let's begin our work here by writing down, in your notebook or the downloaded workbook pages, "I am learning to manage my stress with grace and flexibility, and uplifting myself though gentle self-care," then sign and date it. I also recommend finding a moment to look in the mirror and lovingly tell yourself of this intention, and why—in your own words— that this is important to you.

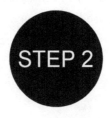

OBSERVE

The next step is pretty simple, but that doesn't mean it is necessarily easy. Step Two is all about active observation. What I mean by that is in this case, try to be as aware as you can of the times you feel a sense of stress overtaking your thoughts and emotions, and write down the magnitude of the types of feelings of stress, how food was involved as a reaction, and other behaviors you noticed. (Of course, in moments of feeling extreme stress you may not have the wherewithal to make notes, so don't worry if you find yourself writing these details down hours—or days—after the fact).

For starters, when you feel stressed, how does it show up physically? Pay attention to what your body is telling you. Do you feel it in your stomach? Or do you get a headache? Maybe you get tense in the shoulders. Some people find it difficult to focus or get lightheaded.

Beyond the physical sensations, it is equally important that you become aware of how you respond to stress through your behavior. Do you eat too much, or too little? Is consuming food a coping mechanism, or does stress have you so upset that you lose your appetite and otherwise ignore good self-care?

Finally, how does being under pressure affect your actions toward the world around you? Do you feel as if stress makes you want to throw things? Lock yourself in your room? Many of us get snippy with the people in our lives when we feel stressed out. Unreleased pressure can lead to feelings of frustration and depression.

Food is one of the most common go-to's used to self-soothe the feelings of stress. Eating may help you feel like you are giving yourself a little TLC, tender loving care. Food also may provide a distraction from whatever it is triggering the stress.

Worksheet #1

We are often not aware of feeling upset until we are so deep into it that the emotion is difficult to manage. So in order to effectively address these feelings of being stressed, it is important to recognize them as they show up. If you can identify these feelings before they run you over, you are more likely to ease them with beneficial coping mechanisms, and can avoid falling into ineffective or dysfunctional activities to self-soothe, like binge eating.

One of the best ways to identify issues that may show up in the future is to observe their characteristics in the past. As you become familiar with previous dynamics of emerging stress, you'll eventually be able to recognize the stress events as they form and then respond in soothing ways to relieve that stress before it all gets out of hand.

I have filled out a sample chart to illustrate what some typical stress events might look like:

	Occurence Date/Time	Approximate Trigger	Sensation	Venting Behavior
Example	Wed. 3/1 9:00PM	Realizing I missed dead- line at work	Feeling of being trapped	Urge to eat rest of ice cream
	Sat. 3/26 11:00AM	In-laws coming to stay during extremely busy week	Overwhelm	Sleeplessness, fatigued in morning, ate more muffins than intended

The person who filled out this chart feels overwhelmed and trapped when stressed. Another person might feel rage, and while someone else might feel like just giving up. The point is, if you are subject to stress-triggered eating, this exercise can help you become attuned to the warning signs, so you can deal with the feelings of stress before they become unmanageable.

Now, it's your turn. Download the Stress Event workbook pages from the "Pressure-Cooker Eater" document in this book's online resource pages, or, to create a Stress Event chart in your notebook, use the sample above as a guide.

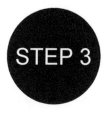

PUTTING STRESS ENERGY TO WORK

As with all problematic eating styles, the solution lies in finding better coping mechanisms.

Let's back up and discuss for a moment stress energy as it rolls around inside. That powerful and uncomfortable energy exists, believe it or not, to help you. It is part of the fight-or-flight mechanism we are all born with. As we discussed in the first part of this book, this energy is instinctual, and is called up when we feel threatened. Animals, for example, will either fight or run in response to their stress energy. But if we are feeling pressure put upon us by our boss, it is not practical or appropriate to get into a physical fight with them or to flee to the hills to alleviate our stress energy.

Additionally, sometimes the feelings of stress are caused by something we cannot deal with at the present moment and must put off to a later time, perhaps a contentious meeting scheduled for later in the week. So you might say that the unutilized fight-or-flight energy gets sort of frustrated. It just swirls around creating feelings of pressure, making us miserable. It is for this reason that I recommend participating in some sort of physical exercise to release the build-up of fight-or-flight energy.

As good as physical activity is, there are also other, non-food ways to alleviate pressure. Channeling your stress energy into being creative or taking time for some targeted self-care can also help soothe feelings of being pressured. I have put together a list of just a few ideas; there are probably many things that would work for you that are not on this list:

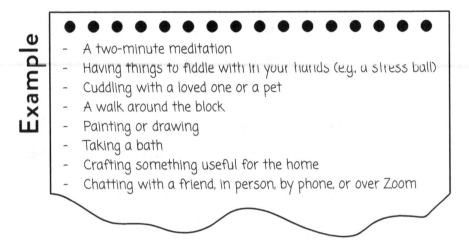

Example

- A two-minute meditation
- Having things to fiddle with in your hands (e.g., a stress ball)
- Cuddling with a loved one or a pet
- A walk around the block
- Painting or drawing
- Taking a bath
- Crafting something useful for the home
- Chatting with a friend, in person, by phone, or over Zoom

(For a more extensive list, see the "Non-Food Ways to Self-Soothe" section in Part Four of this book.)

Worksheet #2 - Non-Food Self-Soothing Techniques

For this exercise, put some thought into non-food things you are able to do to vent your stress energy. You can make a list in your notebook or download Worksheet #2 from the website. You might select some of the items listed above, or come up with some of your own. Make your list as long as possible, and then make a shorter list of the things you like best and can have prepared to enjoy at a moment's notice, whenever you start to feel stressed out.

Ideally, just looking at your list can give you warm feelings of comfort.

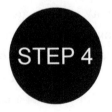

STEP 4

CHALLENGING OLD BEHAVIORS

Let's take stock of how stress is subject to behavior. Are there things you might have done to lessen your stress *before* it had a chance to build?

Becoming aware of where you might be accountable in creating your own stress-triggers is a critical first step towards easing stress...and easing stress-triggered eating!

For example, are you feeling stressed about an assignment because you left it till the last minute? Perhaps adapting better time management skills would be an important strategy for lessening the pressure you feel. Working towards good time management skills is just one way to ease the pressure before it starts. So is developing the ability to renegotiate personal obligations. Learning not to take negative feedback personally (to the point that you beat yourself up over it) is, for some people, a major way not to take on stress. And, as you've probably figured out, there are so

many other ways to reduce stress before it becomes a problem.

Worksheet #3

In your notebook or downloaded "Pressure-Cooker Eater" workbook document, make a list of things that have recently made you feel stressed-out. Then next to each item, make a note describing a strategy that might have made that incident feel less stressful.

Examples:

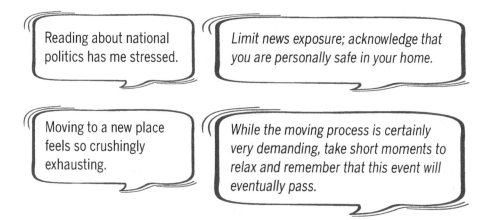

Reading about national politics has me stressed.

Limit news exposure; acknowledge that you are personally safe in your home.

Moving to a new place feels so crushingly exhausting.

While the moving process is certainly very demanding, take short moments to relax and remember that this event will eventually pass.

Now it's your turn. Take your time, you don't need to complete it all in one sitting. After you've made your list, you'll be ready for Step Five.

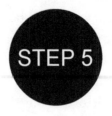

TRANSFORMING STRESS-TRIGGERED EATING RESPONSES

In the previous sections we've discussed how to build awareness of escalating stress...strategies for coping with stress...and that being accountable for what causes you stress can guide you to ways to soften that stress before it becomes unmanageable.

Finally, let's put these important elements together to address stress-triggered eating. Let's say you have a demanding job and you're feeling run-of-the-mill stress and pressure from work. The truth is, that same pressure will be there whether you eat some donuts or an apple—whether you take a walk around the block or walk to the vending machine, do some deep breathing or help yourself to something deep-fried. Managing the stress is really about the response you meet the stress with. And that response is completely your choice.

The difference is that—as we discussed in Step Three: Putting Stress Energy to Work—a walk around the block will allow you to blow off some steam, making it easier to deal with whatever stress you are feeling. A trip to the vending machine may leave you with feelings of sadness and disappointment for not following your eating intentions.

Worksheet #4

The previous exercise explored things in our world that can potentially raise our stress levels. In this exercise, we are turning our attention to specific events.

You'll be working with a chart made up of two columns. In the first column, make note of incidents in which stress has shown up in your life, and how you responded. In the second column, write down an alternate way you might have responded that would have better served you. Here is an example:

	What I Did	What Might Better Serve Me
Example	When my boss was annoyed at me for missing a deadline, I ate a candy bar.	I admit to myself that I could have started the project earlier, or discussed renegotiating the deadline. I make a commitment to myself to be more prepared next time, and do my best to live up to it.
	On a very long Wednesday, I felt so pressured from work, social obligations, and family responsibilities, I finished a pint of ice cream over the sink at midnight.	As soon as I find a moment for quiet at the end of my busy day, I relax with a cup of herbal tea, do some mindful breathing, and focus on all the things I'm grateful for.

Now, it's your turn. In your notebook or workbook pages, fill in your own details in your worksheet.

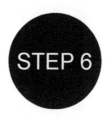

STEP 6

AFFIRM WHO YOU ARE

Finally, as you shift your relationship with stress and with stress-triggered eating, celebrate and take ownership of your new mindful approach. In your notebook or workbook, write down the following statement, putting your name in the provided blank space.:

I am _____. My heart is open, my attitude is flexible, and I gracefully experience my days with gratitude and calm, facing any challenges with integrity and accountability.

You may find it helpful to repeat this affirmation at those times when you feel at all stressed. Remember to read it to yourself each morning for at least a full month (though making it a habit for many more months is recommended.)

12

THE PROCRASTIN-EATER

One of the most common types of "problem" eater I see falls into the category that tends to use food as a distraction. Very often, this eating issue shows up in combination with another issue or two, and I recommend each issue be addressed one at a time.

THE PROCRASTIN-EATER

The *Procrastin-Eater* is a fun term we use for a not-so-fun habit, that of using food to procrastinate and avoid some undesirable chore. And, truth be told, some people also use eating something as a way to put off starting a task or project they actually want to do, but don't really know where or how to start.

This category is such a common one that you would be hard-pressed to find someone who has never decided to eat something as an avoidance excuse at least once in a while. It is certainly not hard to understand; I mean, who wouldn't rather eat a hot-fudge sundae than clean out the garage? Another version of this profile is that some people decide to take a treat reward *before* they start the big project. While I don't recommend using food either as an avoidance technique or as a reward, I certainly understand its appeal.

This turns into a larger problem for some individuals when they use food as the go-to coping mechanism whenever they are faced with a tough task.

Meet Rachel, a 24-year-old graduate student who currently spends most days working on her thesis. She arrived at my office wearing an outfit that suggested she had put some thought into it, and her make-up was tastefully and skillfully applied. Since beginning college, Rachel explained, she had gained a significant amount of weight. Now working toward her Master's degree, she had decided she was ready to commit to some healthful lifestyle changes. She visited my office after beginning her last semester of school, assuming her thesis would be completed by the end of the term. She tearfully spoke of her frustrations with using food as a way of putting off other tasks. She'd think about starting to work, then feel the need to put a snack together, finish the snack, start working for a little while before having something else to eat...in fact, she would snack continuously, and end up feeling physically uncomfortable. Her distress, she explained, came from feeling so inefficient in approaching schoolwork as much as she felt distressed by her seemingly uncontrollable snacking.

Not all people who procrastinate are perfectionists. Some find themselves feeling that they can't manage their time properly, and succumb to a sort of paralysis that comes with not knowing what to do. Others will ignore a project until it is almost too late, needing the urgency of a short deadline to focus their energies in a useful way. I have seen all types use food for task avoidance.

The concept of *mindfulness* and *living mindfully* shows up regularly in my consultation room and in this book, and for good reason. Mindfulness helps us transcend those things that get in our way and keep us from creating the life/circumstances/ways-of-being we would prefer. For our purposes here, applying mindfulness helps with procrastination because being mindful keeps us focused on the specific steps in front of us. Most people get a bit overwhelmed when they try to wrap their minds around major projects or weighty tasks, often getting bogged down just thinking about the most confusing, difficult, or emotionally challenging aspects, resulting in procrastination. Since putting ourselves in a mindful frame of mind keeps us aware of immediate action steps to take *now* —and away from distractions —it's easier to get done what needs to get done without hiding behind a snack.

In Rachel's case, we discussed the pressure she was putting on herself to achieve excellence, and her gnawing anxiety that she would not hit that mark. I did not need to explain to her that most of her procrastination stems from a fear of failure.

I suggested she take time out to be mindful of her goals and her fears, and to be kind with herself. I explained that though her eating and procrastination seemed to be interconnected, they were two separate issues that were—pardon the pun—feeding off of each other. I helped her design a daily schedule around her academics. We built in well-balanced meals with adequate protein and added regularly structured snacks to the schedule —taking care that she make sure she was not hungry before starting any task —to separate and address both elements of her work vs. food dynamic.

And last—but by no means least —another critical feature that we added was some enjoyable "self-care" time (e.g., a bubble-bath), so she could reward herself for working hard during the day with something other than food.

Self-Correction Toolkit for the Procrastin-Eater

To gain the greatest benefit from this toolkit, I highly recommend you obtain a dedicated notebook to do your work in, or download our toolkit worksheets by visiting www.whydidijusteatthat.com/resources and click on the "Procrastin-Eater" link for printable copies.

Oddly enough, though food plays a central role in this issue, the dynamic at play here is largely about procrastination. There are many reasons people procrastinate. Some procrastinators are perfectionists. Others feel so chronically overwhelmed that adding another task to their list is just too stressful. Some people procrastinate as a way to rebel from what they feel is an overly structured or authoritarian environment. (As I mentioned at the beginning of this section, there are usually other eating issues accompanying this one. In my experience, those issues often feed into the core reasons that trigger the procrastinating behaviors.) With that in mind, the strategies we'll be discussing to resolve this issue will focus as much on managing procrastination as it will be on food.

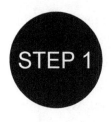

ADMIT...THEN COMMIT

Write a Starting-Point Affirmation

Admit that you understand, for your highest good, that there needs to be a change in your style of thinking. Take some quiet time to acknowledge this, then record your thoughts in your notebook or the downloaded workbook pages. You might write down, "I am committed to disconnecting eating from procrastination and taking greater initiative in doing my tasks," in the space marked Affirmations below, then sign and date it. I also recommend finding a moment to look in the mirror and tell yourself of this intention, and why—in your own words—that this is important to you.

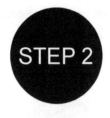

OBSERVE

Observe the number of times this week that you use food in place of finishing a task. Observe it in a non-critical "just noticing" sort of way. Make a list of observations in your notebook or downloaded workbook pages.

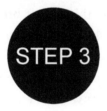

REWORK AND REFRAME

The "Procrastin-eater" describes a convoluted issue because there are really two issues at play here. One issue is about habitually relying on food as a way to avoid tasks, and the other issue is about habitually avoiding tasks. In this scenario, the use of food is a way to self-soothe the sense

of discomfort that arises while facing unpleasant tasks. The "Procrastin-eater" is using food as a reward for completing something...without actually completing it.

Reframing Exercise

So first, let's ignore the procrastination aspect and simply separate food from the equation. In your notebook or downloaded workbook pages, make a list of things you could have done in place of eating; a list of distractions that you might do if you decide to take a break instead of using food.

These things might include taking your dog for a fifteen-minute walk, or meditating for ten minutes, or putting on some music and dancing for ten minutes, or pleasure-reading a chapter in a book. Feel free to come up with your own non-food soothing activity!

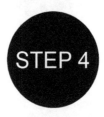

CHALLENGING OLD BEHAVIORS, UNHELPFUL INNER VOICES, ETC.

Once you've found some things that bring you soothing energy and comfort, it is time to begin shifting the emphasis from using these things for avoidance to enjoying them as rewards. If there are small activities that you can use as brief break respites during the completion of tasks, think of pleasant non-food rewards that you can enjoy after your task is finished.

Examples of these might be taking a bubble bath, or getting a manicure, creating a fun craft or art project, or watching a good movie. For a more extensive list of potential rewards, see the "Non-Food Ways to Self-Soothe" section in Part Four of this book.

Now write your ideas for your own Task Completion Rewards in your notebook or downloaded workbook pages!

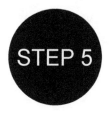

STEP 5

AFFIRM WHO YOU ARE

Behavioral issues take some time to untangle. There are complex reasons behind the habit of procrastination, and it is not likely that these pages completely resolved that issue. What I hope we were able to do is add a little insight to the dynamics of procrastinating behavior—awareness can begin the first steps of progress—and I hope we removed food as part of the avoidance equation.

Obviously, a big part of shifting behavior and expanding comfort levels rests in mindset. We opened this section with an affirmation of intent, and now we'll close this chapter with an affirmation of acknowledgment and centering. This final step is an ongoing process to take firm ownership of a new perspective on how to interact with your world.

In your notebook or workbook, write down the following statement, putting your name in the provided blank space.

> I am _____. I am gentle with myself as I take on tasks, allowing breaks and accepting rewards as part of the process. I sooth myself with activities I enjoy, and savor food in its proper place as joyful nourishment.

Repeat it to yourself every day in quiet moments, perhaps as you lie in bed in the morning or at the end of your day, or while meditating or exercising. Try to do this every day for at least a month. If you forget, that's fine, just forgive yourself and pick up where you left off. Even if you feel uncomfortable or don't fully believe this statement at first, remember that in order to grow, we must become clear on what we aspire to be.

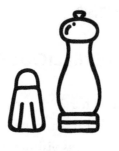

13

THE REBELLIOUS EATER

One aspect common to people in the Rebellious Eater category is that they use food as a form of communication. They tend to consume food—or restrict their intake of food—as a way to say, "I control my body" when so much else seems beyond their control. Rebellious Eaters may eat as a way to express feelings for which they have no words, or don't feel they have the power in their lives to honestly speak the words they do have.

Many people who feel that they have little or no control over important aspects of their lives will employ their use of food as the one facet of their existence they actually have sway over. In a way, food can serve as a method of communication. For example, many people who find it difficult to verbally communicate their anger may use food as a way of expressing I am angry! For them, food comes as a way to demonstrate personal power, a method of silent and passive protest that ends up being self-destructive, because those who use eating as a way to communicate often end up feeling powerless over food.

THE REBELLIOUS EATER

Nicole had just celebrated her 19th birthday and after years of struggling with food issues, decided it was time to commit to healing herself. One of the first steps she took was visiting my office. She explained that her dad's sister was living in a very large body. Nicole's mom was obsessed with being thin —which she held as a core value —and introduced diet rules to Nicole at the age of six, so that she didn't "end up looking like her Aunt Rosie."

Nicole said, "I remember being at the after-school playground I was in second grade, and all the other kids were eating cookies but me. My baby-sitter gave me an apple, I guess on instructions from my mom, and told me that I should eat fruit because it was less fattening. I wasn't even overweight, but it started me feeling that I was."

And so began Nicole's weight and body image struggle. "I didn't want to look like my oversized aunt," she continued, "and began to try to please everyone with my weight...except me." In high school, Nicole went away to a three-week summer weight loss camp, determined to lose as much weight as she could, mostly to please her mother. Coming home nearly 16 pounds lighter, she expected her mom would be thrilled with her results. But to her surprise, "I was met with, 'You look good but you could still stand to lose a little bit more around your waist.'"

That, for Nicole, was the last straw. She felt like there was no pleasing her mom and so fell into a cycle of rebellious eating, thinking, *I'll show you*...and started devouring everything in sight, ultimately gaining almost four times more pounds than she had lost.

One time, Nicole and her mother were at a friend's home when they were offered dessert. Nicole really wanted to have some, but as the plate came around, her mother said, "WE don't want any." Nicole went home and, after her parents had gone to bed, ate an entire box of cookies, thinking, *I'll show her...*

After over a year of this behavior, she felt lost and stuck and hopeless, and that's when she came to me for help.

To start our working together, I encouraged Nicole to take ownership of her own body. I asked who got to decide her body's size and nourishment level. As she began to assume authority over her own body, she began to pay closer attention to her hunger and fullness cues. We talked about what it meant for her to honor her body, and she started to look at the self-care of her body as a way to celebrate it.

(There's a surprising sidenote to this one. Nicole had been so intimidated by her sense of her mother's inflexibility she had assumed that to bring her mom to one of our sessions would be fruitless. After several sessions, as she began to feel stronger, she finally did agree to invite her mom, Betsy, to join us for a session, so Nicole could share her feelings. Betsy was surprised to hear what Nicole had to share, and was able to accept responsibility for her part in contributing to Nicole's eating disorder. It turned out that she had herself been struggling with age-related issues regarding her own body, and was beginning to question her own assumptions about how women's bodies should look. She apologized to her daughter for her insensitivity, and this brought the two women closer; each of them committed to improving their health and now both even go to the gym together!)

Self-Correction Toolkit for the Rebellious Eater

To gain the greatest benefit from this toolkit, I highly recommend you obtain a dedicated notebook to do your work in, or download our toolkit worksheets by visiting www.whydidijusteatthat.com/resources and click on the "Rebellious Eater" link for printable copies.

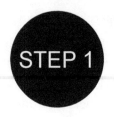

STEP 1

ADMIT...THEN COMMIT

Rebellious eating is rooted in a sense of powerlessness—against a life situation, against a person, against food itself. So the first step is to begin to assert your power.

Write a Starting-Point Affirmation

Admit that you understand, for your highest good, that there needs to be a change in your mindset regarding your personal agency. Take some quiet time to acknowledge this, then record your thoughts in your notebook or the downloaded workbook pages. You might write down, "I am moving toward asserting more control over the things in my life that are important to me," in the space marked Affirmations below, then sign and date it. I also recommend finding a moment to look in the mirror and tell yourself of this intention, and why—in your own words—that this is important to you.

NUTRITION BYTE: It is unfortunate that it is easier for some people to give others the benefit of the doubt than to offer themselves any kindness. While even thoughts of embracing active self-kindness may make some people uncomfortable, this is one case where a fake-it-till-you-make-it strategy is super important!

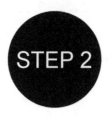

OBSERVE

Oftentimes, when we are used to certain behaviors—including our behaviors that we don't like or don't serve us—it is a challenge to be aware of them, even as we are doing them. So take your time, and simply try to notice the things that trigger you emotionally. We are especially interested in those instances that you respond to by emotionally triggered eating or restricting.

Observe the occasions you're feeling angry, frustrated, or upset and food becomes your go-to instead of using your voice. Keep track of these incidents on this workbook page, or open a list app in your smartphone, tablet, or computer. Take your time with this process and be gentle with yourself if you identify trends about your behavior that you realize you don't like.

Examples of Rebellious-Eater behaviors you might observe in yourself might look like these:

"When my boss sticks me with a huge job at the last minute, I have to take a break and have a big plate of comfort food, even though I feel bad after eating it."

"When my husband ignores my preferences, it's easier for me to go eat something, rather than make it a thing."

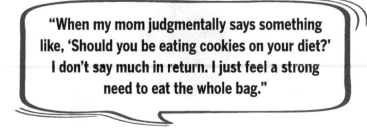

"When my mom judgmentally says something like, 'Should you be eating cookies on your diet?' I don't say much in return. I just feel a strong need to eat the whole bag."

Activity: Collect Your Own Observations of Your Rebellious-Eater Behaviors

Spend a week or so watching and recording your responses and reactions to these triggers until you see patterns emerge. You can use the workbook pages you downloaded from this book's website, or make a section in your notebook to track your experiences. Then go on to Step Three.

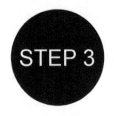

STEP 3

REWORK AND REFRAME

In Step Two, you made some notes describing instances when you responded to certain triggers through food. Are there any conclusions you are able to observe?

For example, in moments of potential conflict, do you find you swallow your responses by eating food, instead of asserting yourself? Or does eating function as a mechanism for you to push your anger down, making you feel somewhat bad about yourself but allowing you to avoid dealing with deeper upset feelings? Do you use eating as a rebellious tactic to get back at some other person, especially if that person is projecting critical judgments over food and what—and how much—food you are eating? Is it possible you rebelliously eat unhealthy food choices as a way to inflict self-harm when you feel bad about yourself? Or is the rebellious-eating dynamic in your case a combination of two or more of these elements?

The irony is that Rebellious Eaters harm themselves more than they harm anyone else. Their actions of rebelliousness speak to a feeling of some level of powerlessness. In the game of rebellion, they are both perpetrator and victim.

The way out of the Rebellious Eater dynamic is simple, but not easy. The way out is to find ways to go from being a victim...to becoming empowered!

Let's look at the examples from Step Two, this time adding more empowering responses:

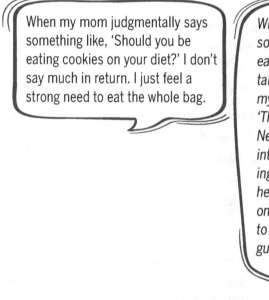

When my mom judgmentally says something like, 'Should you be eating cookies on your diet?' I don't say much in return. I just feel a strong need to eat the whole bag.

When my mom judgmentally says something like, 'Should you be eating cookies in your diet?' I take a moment to check in with my feelings and then say to her, 'Thank you for caring about me. Nevertheless, monitoring my intake is my job, and I'm learning what works for me. When I hear other people commenting on my intake, it's hard for me to listen to my own internal guidance.'

Some people are reluctant to assert themselves with their parents because they do not want to seem like they are disrespecting their mom or dad. But ideally, we should make all of our communications—especially those in which we stand up for ourselves—with respect for everyone, including ourselves. There is no guarantee, of course, that the mom in this scenario would be able to really understand what is being said, but the simple act of speaking your mind and using your voice may help you regain a sense of personal power and alleviate that awful feeling of not being heard.

(As a side note, it is not unusual for a Rebellious Eater to have been raised by an "All-or-Nothing Eater." To understand a little something about that eater, check out Chapter 1.)

Now, let's look at the next example:

> When my boss sticks me with a huge job at the last minute, I have to take a break and have a big plate of comfort food, even though I feel bad after eating it.

> *When my boss sticks me with a huge job at the last minute, I acknowledge to myself that I feel frustrated and at the first opportunity I will treat myself with kindness in a non-food way. For instance, I might go home and have a hot bath and listen to music that I like.*

Sometimes it is inappropriate to express to someone (in this case, a boss) that you are upset over a decision that involves you. Even so, it is important to acknowledge and validate your own feelings to yourself—and beyond that—develop ways to soothe upset feelings other than eating for comfort. Finally, let's look at the third example:

> When my husband ignores my preferences, it's easier for me to go eat something, rather than get into an argument with him.

> *When my husband ignores my preferences, I can state my truth without being combative, and calmly share with him that I feel frustrated when my preferences are ignored.*

Using an "I" statement is a good way for us to stand up for our own needs without making the other person wrong. Using the word "You" in a statement like this could easily be perceived as accusatory, even if that is not the intention. In an "I" statement, we describe and take responsibility for our own feelings without ascribing motives or criticisms to the other person.

In all of these cases and in any others, one of the most empowering things we can do is take a moment to access our feelings when we feel an emotional challenge coming on. First, we look inward and ask, what is the feeling, and what might be causing it? Then, as is appropriate, calmly discuss it with the relevant people involved in the situation.

Activity: Re-examine Your Own Behaviors

Step Three Exercise: Now that you've had a chance to consider my three examples of empowering responses, it's your turn. Review the observations of your personal instances of rebellious eater behaviors that you noted in Step Two of the exercises. Then, in your notebook or workbook pages, write down your own empowering responses to each of these observations.

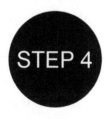

STEP 4

PRACTICE AWARENESS

Over time and through dedicated introspection, old "Rebellious-Eater habits" will soon become easy to identify even before they fully surface. (The challenge is, of course, that they tend to surface during emotionally triggering moments.) In these situations, with awareness and gentleness toward yourself, focus on taking a moment to check in with your feelings. Then take another moment to use your voice.

Activity: Plan Ahead for Your Emotion Triggers

Reflect each morning how you are planning to deal with the emotion triggers that might urge you to eat. Reflect each evening how you respond during that day. Visualizing standing up for yourself is a great tool to support these reflections. Do this each day until it is second nature. Be patient and flexible. No need to try to be perfect; good enough is good enough.

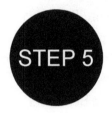

AFFIRM WHO YOU ARE

We opened these exercises with an affirmation of intent, and now we'll close this chapter with an affirmation of acknowledgement and centering. This final step is an ongoing process to take firm ownership of a new perspective on how to interact with your world.

In your notebook or workbook, write down the following statement, putting your name in the provided blank space.

> I am _____. My open heart empowers me to speak my truth, as I take care of myself and share my loving energy with those in my life. I am enough, and worthy just as I am now.

Try to repeat your new affirmation to yourself every day in quiet moments, perhaps as you lie in bed in the morning or at the end of your day, or while meditating or exercising. Try to do this every day for at least a month. If you forget, that's fine, just forgive yourself and pick up where you left off. Even if you don't fully believe this statement at first, remember that in order to grow, we must become clear on what we aspire to be.

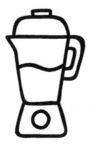

14

THE SEE-FOOD EATER

Despite our little play on words, this type of eater is not someone who enjoys food sourced from the ocean. (That would be the "Seafood Eater.") I identify the See-Food Eater as someone who often feels prompted to eat simply by being exposed to available, tempting food items. What makes some people find the very sight of something appetizing compelling enough to impulsively want to eat that item, even if they are already full from a previous meal? I don't think we can underestimate the role that our senses—sight and smell, and even the sound of food sizzling—play in our appetite and our desire for food.

THE SEE-FOOD EATER

You know that old joke about the guy on the "seafood diet?" (Punchline: "I *see* food; I eat it.") For too many people, that pretty much sums up their eating strategies.

Janet, a 52-year-old single mom, sat perplexed in my office. She was trying to understand why, the night before, she had eaten the plate of chocolate chip cookies sitting on the kitchen counter even though she was actually very full from the ample-sized dinner she had eaten earlier that evening. We discussed the body's hunger and fullness cues, particularly focusing on how the fullness cue works and what, if anything, would make her override these cues.

Janet admitted that seeing appealing food would instantly make her crave the item, lamenting that it was almost as if her eyes had a hunger scale of their own! "I may be full, but once I see it, I want it," she said. For many visually triggered eaters, the visual cue of food—especially enticing, super-palatable foods—can trump the satiety cue. While it might be a good idea to minimize the visual availability of such enticing delicacies to avoid temptation, the larger issue at hand is to learn how to bypass the visually triggered desire and improve our ability to honor our body's cues.

There are all sorts of reasons that allow visual cues to overpower satiety cues. For one thing, hunger cues are obvious ones; they take the form of discomfort in our stomachs, telling us we need nutrition. The sense of being excessively full, on the other hand, is a feeling of discomfort of having more food than necessary in our stomachs. But the middle-ground feeling of being satiated, that is, no longer hungry, is much subtler; in the hunger/fullness sense it is really an *absence* of discomfort. So as cues go, this is one that is pretty easy to ignore.

And there are a lot of elements that cause us to ignore the fact that we are not hungry. As we will discuss in "Chapter 15, The Sleep-Deprived Snacker," sleep deprivation makes it harder to form and follow positive eating strategies. Elevated levels of stress and anxiety can also compromise our commitment to making the best self-care decisions for ourselves.

I asked Janet what it might be like for her if she were to put any enticing leftovers or coveted sweets into lidded containers and put them away in the freezer, fridge, or inside cabinets or drawers, in order to set-up a kind of "out-of-sight, out-of-mind" approach. As in the case of so many other eating struggles, the first step in dealing with getting past playing the part of the "See-Food Eater" is an awareness that there actually is some behavior in need of shifting, and the follow up is taking preventative steps to alleviate situations that might bring about these unwanted behaviors.

Self-Correction Toolkit for the See-Food Eater

> To gain the greatest benefit from this toolkit, I highly recommend you obtain a dedicated notebook to do your work in, or download our toolkit worksheets by visiting www.whydidijusteatthat.com/resources and click on the "See-Food Eater" link for printable copies.

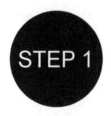

STEP 1

ADMIT...THEN COMMIT

Write a Starting-Point Affirmation

Admit that you understand, for your highest good, that there needs to be a change in your approach to food consumption. Take some quiet time to acknowledge this, then record your thoughts in your notebook or the downloaded workbook pages. You might write down, "I am opening myself up to creating a healthy relationship with food and accepting awareness of what my body is experiencing and what it needs," in the space marked Affirmations below, then sign and date it. I also recommend finding a moment to look in the mirror and tell yourself of this intention, and why—in your own words—that this is important to you.

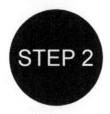

OBSERVE

"See-food" eating might also be called "sensory-triggered impulsive eating." See-food eaters often perceive something appealing—perhaps the smell of chocolate cookies fresh from the oven, or the sight of leftover French fries, or seeing platters of small hors d'oeuvres at a party—and impulsively help themselves to a generous portion of the food that has caught their attention.

The first step toward shifting unwanted behavior toward more beneficial conduct is to become aware of the behavior that isn't serving us. Often, the old behavior has become so familiar we don't even notice it. So our first step is simple observation.

Activity: Record Impulsive Eating

In your notebook or workbook pages, keep track of the times you find yourself impulsively eating foods you happen to see outside of meal or snack time. A few examples of this might be:

- Complimentary donuts in an office breakroom
- Leftovers you come across while clearing the table
- An overabundance of food samples at Costco or the food market

It is possible that it won't occur to you that you are impulsively being a See-Food Eater until well after you have eaten the food you came across; after all, part of being a See-Food Eater is not giving what you are eating much thought. It is okay if—as you start to make a list of See-Food Eating occasions—you start out by noting things that happened days, or even weeks ago. The point is to pull this unconscious habit into your awareness so that this dynamic is more present in your mind.

Activity: Analyze Your Impulsive Eating

In the previous exercise you made a list of "See-Food" events. As you have been giving the matter thought and have become more aware of this dynamic, you may have noticed that you wrote down a few more "See-Food" events than you had expected to at first. In this next step, consider your desire to have each item, listing all the reasons why eating that item seems like a good idea. And then, following that, challenge the idea of eating these foods with reasons why it isn't such a good idea.

Based on the previous examples, a few examples might be:

Example

Complimentary donuts in an office break room.
Reason to eat what you see: donuts taste good.
Reasons challenging eating the donuts: • Eating when you aren't hungry goes against health goals. • Your body might not feel great after eating donuts if you're too full. • Eating the donut might make you want to skip a more nutritious lunch.

Leftovers you come across while clearing the table.
Reason to eat what you see: • The food tastes good. • Eating left-overs is easier than putting them away.
Reasons challenging eating the leftovers: • Eating after a meal has ended may make you over-full. • You can enjoy the leftovers at another meal when you are hungry- and would appreciate them more at that time.

An overabundance of food samples at Costco or the food market.
Reason to eat what you see: • The samples look appealing. • There are opportunities to taste foods new to you.
Reasons challenging eating what you see: • Your body doesn't feel great after eating so much food, even if it • comes in small servings it still adds up. • Grazing on tons of store samples isn't a terribly healthy meal. • Having a taste of a new-to-you food is probably fine (unless you are • allergic to the sample,) but eating a lot of stuff already familiar to you • simply because it is there goes against health goals. • Eating when you aren't hungry also goes against health goals.

You will have your own listed items, of course, and your own reasons to eat these items...as well as reasons not to. You may find that in most cases, the reasons not to be a "See-Food" Eater are more substantial than the reason to impulse eat. Using either your downloaded workbook pages or your notebook, make note of your own reasons to eat what you see, and then reasons challenging eating what you see.

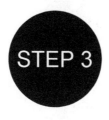

EMBRACE INTUITIVE EATING

If you are working the steps in this chapter, you probably understand why it is best not to habitually be an impulsive "See-Food" Eater. Yet, spotting a tray of hot chocolate chip cookies freshly out of the oven will probably seem appealing to most people. How are some people able to resist such temptations while others find fighting the impulse to eat it much more challenging?

The answer is that many people have found a way to rise above unwanted eating habits through intuitive eating.

Intuitive eating can best be described as a non-dieting approach to eating strategies. Its purpose is to help people let go of rule-based approaches to eating while eating in more flexible manners. Our bodies have an innate wisdom. If we can only learn to listen to what our bodies call for, we can follow eating practices that satisfy our nutrition needs.

One important step toward becoming an intuitive eater is to become fully aware of our hunger and fullness cues. I suggest thinking of these cues in the context of a hunger/fullness meter, a scale that measures the range of sensations from feeling hungry to feeling full in increments of 1 to 10, with "1" being super hungry and "10" feeling overly full.

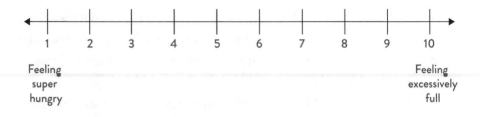

Feeling
super
hungry

Feeling
excessively
full

I define intuition as instinct in action. Not bound by rules, eating intuitively is all about us listening to our own bodies, separate from "shoulds" and rules. When we follow this approach, our bodies dictate when we are hungry and when it's time to stop eating. When we let go of eating-related "shoulds," there is no right or wrong connected to our relationships with food and eating. (For a deeper dive into the dynamics and benefits of eating intuitively, please check out my thoughts in Chapter 5, The Fad-Food Eater.)

So let's get back to that tray of freshly baked cookies we were discussing at the start of this section. At the sight of the cookies, intuitive eaters will understand a few things:

 They know that if they eat an abundance of cookies (or an abundance of anything for that matter) they will not feel so good.

 An intuitive eater will know that if they really want a cookie they can eat it; they can eat it now, they can eat it later, or tomorrow, or next week. They will understand that since they can have it whenever, they don't have to eat a cookie right now. They can eat the cookie when it feels right to do so. The intuitive sense of their body is in charge.

 The intuitive eating approach to food is flexible and conceived not to be perfect, but to be good enough.

The exercise for Step 3 is to check in with your body at every meal and snack. Put a reminder in your phone to have *mindful meals* in which you consider how your mind and body and spirit react to foods as you eat. Eat slowly. And don't forget to feel grateful for the effort all along the food production and fulfillment chain that brings the food to your plate.

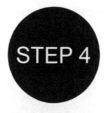

STEP 4

CHALLENGING OLD BEHAVIORS, UNHELPFUL INNER VOICES, ETC.

This final step will put your work connecting with intuitive eating to practical use. What I am about to suggest may seem like a crazy assignment, but just remember...you don't need to do it out loud!

Activity: Address Your Impulsive Eating

Every time you find yourself in a "See-Food" situation—that is, whenever you find yourself enticed to impulsively eat something—have a conversation with your body:

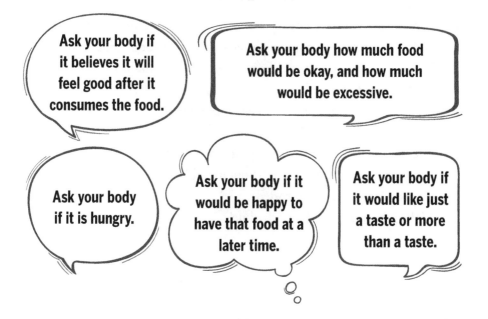

You might have this conversation written out like a play, or as a silent conversation in your mind. In the beginning this exercise may feel uncomfortable, but its benefit will become apparent in no time. Eventually, you won't even have to have this conversation, your body will supply you with intuition-based answers before you even ask the questions.

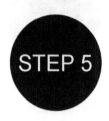

STEP 5

AFFIRM WHO YOU ARE

We began these exercises with a statement of acknowledgment, and we'll end with an affirmation—lock in your new eating strategy by celebrating and making this statement your own. In your notebook or workbook, write down the following statement, putting your name in the provided blank space.:

> I am _____. I have power over choices of whether to eat or not and I eat intuitively, enjoying a wide variety of foods that feed my body and soul. I trust and honor my body's intuition in knowing what is best for it.

It can be very effective to repeat your affirmation to yourself each morning for at least a full month (though making it a habit for many more months is certainly recommended).

Make it part of your daily schedule!

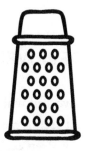

15

THE SLEEP-DEPRIVED SNACKER

I wasn't very far into my practice when I realized just how many people use food as a way to compensate for inadequate sleep. Practicing sensible sleep habits is a critical way to maintain good health—we all know that—yet too often we simply don't get enough shut-eye. We might have too much to do, or perhaps we allow ourselves a few too many moments to decompress at the end of a long day, or maybe it's just the problem of time sort of getting away from us and before we know it we're in bed later than we had originally planned.

Unfortunately, sleep cannot be banked; that is, you cannot get too little sleep all week, and then stock up on it on weekends. The effects of being chronically sleep-deprived carry on for quite a while.

THE SLEEP-DEPRIVED SNACKER

Charlie was a 64-year-old divorced male who had a great deal of difficulty sleeping. When he started seeing me, his best estimate was that he was averaging about five hours of sleep each night. He reported that each morning he would roll out of bed tired and then bang down around four cups of coffee to "wake (himself) up." He told me that he would generally function okay at work, until 3:00 p.m. when an afternoon lull would hit him and he'd find himself growing sleepy. To wake himself up, he would take as many as three trips to the vending machine for candy or other high-calorie snacks, just to make it through the rest of his workday.

The first recommendation I made to Charlie was to suggest he have a sleep study. Sure enough, he was diagnosed with a significant case of sleep apnea, which was dramatically impacting his sleep. Charlie began using a C-PAP machine and his night's sleep improved dramatically, literally overnight. His daily vending machine trips decreased from three to two and then dwindled down to one. Within a few weeks, Charlie was able to completely eliminate this habit, and ultimately replaced the candy bars with a snack (higher in protein and fiber) that he brought from home.

Poor sleep habits have a direct connection to poor eating habits. There may be multiple reasons for this. One study's findings implies that during the times we don't get enough sleep, we are liable to eat more food than usual to take in extra energy to help our lagging bodies stay awake.[3] Moreover, when food is easily accessible, tired people tend to eat even more than is actually required.

It could be that when we are continually tired, our self-discipline is weaker than when we are fully rested. Studies suggest that because the brain functions required to think complex decisions through are dulled, fatigued people might make less-than-optimum choices.[4] Sleep deprivation is no friend of good cognitive functioning!

Sleep deprivation leads to changes in thermoregulation; in other words, some people feel chilly when they don't get enough sleep. These people may crave additional calories to burn for additional warmth. (The process of burning calories to keep warmth is called *thermogenesis*.)

Moreover, the brains of sleepy people have high levels of 2-arachidonoylglycerol, or 2-AG, a brain chemical very much like a chemical found in cannabis. In other words, being sleep-deprived might very well be giving us the munchies!

While it is not unusual to need a little snack in the middle of the afternoon, being chronically sleep-deprived can feed cravings that lead to unhealthy choices. The best thing we all can do, obviously, is make sure to get enough sleep! Sometimes missing out on enough sleep is unavoidable; in those cases I recommend preparing healthy food portions ahead of time so if the "drowsy cravings" strike, you don't have to rely on tempting poor snack choices.

Self-Correction Toolkit for the Sleep-Deprived Snacker

To gain the greatest benefit from this toolkit, I highly recommend you obtain a dedicated notebook to do your work in, or download our toolkit worksheets by visiting www.whydidijusteatthat. com/resources and click on the "Sleep-Deprived Snacker" link for printable copies.

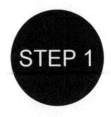

ADMIT...THEN COMMIT

Write a Starting-Point Affirmation

Admit that you understand, for your highest good, that there needs to be a change in your style of thinking. Take some quiet time to acknowledge this, then record your thoughts in your notebook or the downloaded workbook pages. You might write down, "I am altering my habits to demonstrate revitalized commitment to myself through improved self-care," in the space marked Affirmations below, then sign and date it. I also recommend finding a moment to look in the mirror and tell yourself of this intention, and why—in your own words—that this is important to you.

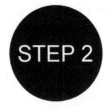

OBSERVE

One major job of our multi-functional brains is to make sure we have enough energy to operate at maximum efficiency. If we are tired (but it's far from bedtime and we can't take a nap), our instinct is often to reach for something to eat; food acts to give us a burst of energy by increasing blood sugar levels. The downside is that eating something does nothing about our actual fatigue level, and when food has been processed, our energy drops again, leaving us feeling even more tired and even more hungry.

In addition to facilitating poor eating habits and food issues, inadequate sleep can lead to mood swings and increased anxiety and can elevate blood pressure. Issues stemming from being a Sleep-Deprived Eater are as much—if not more—about sleep-related self-care as they are about eating-related self-care.

Start by asking yourself, "Why am I getting so little sleep?" Is the problem physical (e.g., sleep apnea, bladder issues) or is it behavior-based? Do you find yourself staying up later than you know you should, just to watch just one more episode of your favorite Netflix show? Do you crawl into bed at a decent time but then stare at your phone until more time than you'd like to admit has flown by?

Activity: Sleep and Food/Mood Diary

Keep a Sleep and Food/Mood Diary for at least a week. Whatever you suspect your sleep-related issues might be, don't commit to any change just yet. Keep the following Sleep and Food/Mood Diary for the next week to get a sense of your relationship with sleep as it currently is. It is critical that you are as honest with the details as possible. After all, we cannot make necessary steps in the right direction if we do not at first know where we stand.

Either download and print the Sleep and Food/Mood Diary from this book's resource pages or copy the following chart in your notebook seven times, one for each day.

Example

Date	Activities you did an hour before bedtime the night before?	Bedtime the night before	Approx. min. to fall asleep the night before	Wake up time	# hours of sleep	Factors affecting sleep the day before (stress, caffeine, sweets, meds etc.)	Write start time and food consumed next to each eating event	Mood and energy/fatigue levels
							Breakfast	
							Mid-morning	
							Late-morning	
							Noon	
							Mid-afternoon	
							Late-afternoon	
							Early evening	
							Late Evening	
							Before bedtime	

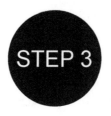

REWORK AND REFRAME

Now that you have filled out your diary, you might begin to make sense of your relationship with sleep.

Activity: Identify Concerns and Determine Solutions in Your Sleep and Food/Mood Diary

If you are getting less than eight hours of slumber, what are you letting be more important than getting a full and adequate night's sleep? Are there activities you engage in just before bedtime that keep you awake?

For example, looking at screens—whether they are smartphones, computer monitors or TV screens—does double duty, in terms of ruining sleep. Not only does interacting with media content serve to stimulate your mind and keep you awake, staring at the light emitted by the screens tends to stimulate one's physiology into not falling asleep.

Some experts recommend turning off lights in your home so the environment is dim and minimally illuminated at least an hour before bedtime. And instead of looking at a screen, consider reading something pleasant and low key by soft, warm lamplight.

Some common items people have noted in their diary are related to what they eat and drink before bed. Consuming too much food before bedtime, for instance, can make you feel uncomfortable and inhibit sleep. Moreover, a full stomach might trigger acid reflux in people who are susceptible, which can lead to other health problems. Carbonated soft drinks, acidic foods, or some sweets containing chocolate may also trigger acid reflux. Drinking beverages containing alcohol may make you sleepy at first but often leads to uncomfortable, non-restful nights. And of course, caffeine before bed is often a culprit in fractured sleep; some people even find their night-time sleep has been disrupted by drinking caffeine beverages in the afternoon, several hours earlier.

Note: In the Case Study at the beginning of this chapter, Charlie reported that he would drink around four cups of coffee to "wake (himself) up." Aside from the minimal nutrition supplied by starting his day with only coffee, coffee can also be an appetite suppressant. That left Charlie extra hungry later in his day!

The solution in these cases is, obviously, to refrain from consuming these foods and drinks beyond an appropriate point in the day.

Some people note an inconsistent sleep schedule regarding bedtimes marked in their diaries. They may observe that they head for bed too late on weekdays—waking before sleeping the recommended eight full hours— and then sleep late on weekends in an attempt to replenish their lost sleep. (Unfortunately, as we mentioned earlier, lost sleep cannot be reacquired, nor can you store sleep hours to make up for lost sleep later.) They may also nap too late in the day, and that is affecting their nighttime sleep.

The truth is that consistent sleep habits are critical to good sleep-related health and such consistency serves to fortify your sleeping/waking cycle. Additionally, there are things you might do to encourage sleep. In addition to dimming the lights, work to keep your sleeping area peaceful and quiet, and keep the temperature at a comfortable level, not too warm or too cool. There are also nutritional steps you might take. Supplements such as melatonin and GABA have been shown to aid in sleep; be sure to consult with your healthcare provider before taking any supplements.

Now look through your diary and take stock of what you have logged in the different sections.

Exercise: Sleep Busters/Sleep Solutions

Either download and print the Sleep Busters/Sleep Solutions chart from this book's resource pages or create a two-column chart in your notebook marked "Sleep Busters" and "Sleep Solutions." Write down issues and items that are keeping you from consistent, healthful sleep in the "Sleep Busters" column. Next to these entries, indicate action steps you can take to improve the situation in the "Sleep Solutions" column. See the example below:

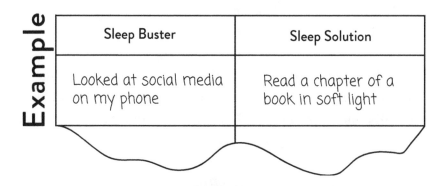

	Sleep Buster	Sleep Solution
Example	Looked at social media on my phone	Read a chapter of a book in soft light

A final note: If you are getting the recommended amount of sleep and still wake up exhausted, perhaps your problem is related to common physical issues. Snoring and sleep apnea, for example, can be obstacles to healthful sleep. (If you sleep with another person within earshot, they will probably let you know if you snore.) If snoring or sleep apnea is the case, perhaps a sleep study is a necessary step toward good sleep. A sleep study may be called for if you are waking up after eight hours of sleep but still feel exhausted. A conversation with your healthcare provider may be in order to follow up these potential problems.

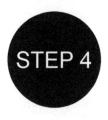

STEP 4

WHAT'S NEXT...

As we discussed earlier in this chapter, the disordered eating stemming from the Sleep-Deprived Eater is as much about sleep (or the lack of) as it is about food and eating habits. Sleep restores your immune system, reboots your body, and cleanses your brain. People who don't get enough sleep tend to eat extra food for energy in compensation, among other reasons.

Honoring your body's need for sleep by resolving the problems identified in the Sleep and Food/Mood Diary should go a long way toward resolving the residual food and eating concerns.

The activity for this section is simply to put the solutions you have written down in the previous exercise to work. As I have frequently pointed out, nobody is perfect at making positive changes all the time, so don't let it get you down or make you give up. What counts is consistent progress; occasional missteps are certainly allowed on the path toward living your best life!

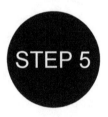

AFFIRM WHO YOU ARE

We opened these exercises with an affirmation of aspiration, and we will close them with one of intention. This final step is an ongoing process to take firm ownership of your more healthful approach to self-care.

In your notebook or workbook, write down the following statement, putting your name in the provided blank space:

> I am _____. I mindfully embrace good self-care and have arranged my life so that I get enough sleep; in doing so I steadily manage my nutrition intake in a healthy manner.

Try to repeat your new affirmation to yourself every day in quiet moments, perhaps as you lie in bed in the morning or at the end of your day, or while meditating or exercising, every day for at least a month.

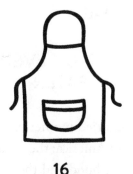

16

THE "TAKING-CARE-OF-EVERYONE-BUT-ME" EATER

Focused on satisfying so many pressing obligations, too many people see simple self-care as somewhat frivolous; a luxury best pushed aside when there are so many immediate issues to attend to. It probably will not come as a surprise to anyone to learn that not allowing time to meet their basic needs tends to leave people feeling depleted, and people that feel depleted may regularly compensate by filling themselves up with food, often without realizing it.

THE "TAKING-CARE-OF-EVERYONE-BUT-ME" EATER

Erica is a 51-year-old married mother of three, and a member of that expanding cohort of modern America: the sandwich generation, caught in between obligations of parenthood and the need to be available to aging parents. She has a husband, a track star daughter who is in her sophomore year in high school, another daughter away at college, and a son who has graduated college and is living at home. She is also trying to make herself as available as she can for her aging mother.

Erica readily admits—with a mixture of pride and resignation—to paying much more attention to the needs of her husband, their children, her mother, and her husband's business, while short-shifting her own needs. Just listening to Erica talk about her day made me want to lie down and take a nap. She supports her husband's asphalt refinishing business by doing his accounting, keeping up on promotion-related correspondence and returning his company's phone calls when he's in the field. She also does all the housework and meal preparation, and drives her daughter to and from meets and track practice. Erica regularly drives a handful of miles away to check in on her mother, often helping with her mom's meals and doing a little gardening for her.

She started seeing me because she had been feeling that her eating was getting out of control. She had no set mealtimes during the day, instead grabbing food here and there when she could. She was pretty good about listening and responding to her body's hunger cues; where she needed help was in making sure the food she did grab was balanced and not just a handful of cookies on her way to the car, or a banana in between laundry loads. She did try to eat dinner with her family, relying mostly on convenience foods and then found herself eating her family's leftovers the next day out of a sense of obligation.

While once upon a time she used to work out by jogging, that part of her life had been just about totally squeezed out due to time constraints. She was feeling uncomfortable in her body, and felt she had lost her way in regard to her own self-care. She wanted to be eating in a way that would fit with her particular uncertain lifestyle, and would still be healthy and—as she put it—efficient. (The idea of efficiency is a trap that I've seen quite a few people—especially women—fall into.)

As we worked together, it was clear that we needed to address two connected aspects of her situation:

1. Her desire for an efficient approach to eating.
2. Her unmet need for self-care.

The efficient part was simple enough to address.

As is the case in so many of the other "eater" categories, preparation often saves the day. Since a lack of free time had her grabbing less nourishing food choices, we thought of ways that she might be prepared for healthy eating and snacking opportunities. For example, just a little extra time at the supermarket reading nutrition labels on packaged foods could result in a freezer stocked with reasonably nutritious meals. Or, once a week she might set up a week's worth of chopped veggies and a tasty dip. Since her kids were clearly old enough, Erica could assign cutting up the vegetables as a regular chore to one of her children. (Kids are busy, but even the busiest kid can pre-wash lettuce or chop some veggies for bulk fridge storage.) Erica might also make extra portions of the nutritious meals she makes for her family in order to have something healthy for herself to eat.

Planning and preparation was also part of the solution in addressing Erica's lack of her own self-care. We first took some time in one of our sessions to acknowledge the need each of us has for self-care, that taking care of ourselves is not a selfish act, but a mindful, self-actualized one. We considered the possibility that, in the times she felt overworked and under-appreciated, she was also under-appreciating *herself*, an attitude that was reflected in her at-times shoddy self-care. And we discussed the truth that, as a practical issue, if she didn't take adequate care of herself, she could run out of emotional/physical/spiritual gas and then crash and burn and be able to take care of *nobody!*

One aspect of good self-care is movement and/or exercise. We discussed the idea that one need not be trapped in the full workout or nothing dynamic. If she craves more exercise, she might find other ways to satisfy the need for movement and keeping her muscles toned. For instance, she could use stairs instead of the elevator, or walk as much as possible, or do push-ups with her toes on the floor and her hands gripping the counter while waiting for coffee in the kitchen, or in the bathroom while waiting for the shower to heat up. Once the desire is acknowledged and the ability to look outside the box is embraced, there are plenty of ways to address a need... even within the constraints of limited time.

To find a way to be more mindful or spiritual, she might spend a few moments planting little weekly or daily alarms in her phone as reminders to take a moment now and then to focus on gratitude or devotional thoughts.

In time, she realized that by acknowledging the need for pre-planning and taking some time to organize her actions, she found she was eating better, felt better cared for, and was happier with her life.

Self-Correction Toolkit for the "Taking-Care-of-Everyone-but-Me" Eater

> To gain the greatest benefit from this toolkit, I highly recommend you obtain a dedicated notebook to do your work in, or download our toolkit worksheets by visiting www.whydidijusteatthat.com/resources and click on the "Taking Care of Everyone but Me" link for printable copies.

It seems that our society has deep-seated expectations and assumptions around how women (in particular, but not always) should be taking care of others at the expense of taking care of themselves. As a result, it is not uncommon for these women to deny their own self-care, which often leads to resentments and frustration from feelings of being neglected. Many of my clients use food as a way of satisfying these feelings of being uncared for. Some are so tired after taking care of everybody else that at the end of the day food becomes their escape, a bright spot after a long day of endless demands. Some people will "numb out" while they eat, disconnected from experiencing the taste, texture, and satisfaction of their food, using it to solve a problem that has nothing to do with nutrition.

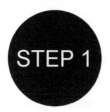

ADMIT...THEN COMMIT

Write a Starting-Point Affirmation

Admit that you understand, for your highest good, that there needs to be a change in your style of thinking. Take some quiet time to acknowledge this, then record your thoughts in your notebook or the downloaded workbook pages. You might write down, "I am willing to open my heart to embrace myself and my needs, taking time to give myself the care that I deserve," in the space marked Affirmations below, then sign and date it. I also recommend finding a moment to look in the mirror and tell yourself of this intention, and why—in your own words—that this is important to you.

> **NUTRITION BYTE:** Making time for a meal is not a reward for satisfying your obligations. Making time for a meal is simply good self-care!

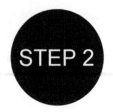

OBSERVE

It is way too easy to lose ourselves and forget about our own needs in the non-stop workload of satisfying our responsibilities for the people in our care; our children, elderly parents, employers, customers, or pets.

Take a moment to observe your role in your various relationships. Does the balance of your interaction with other people involve putting in an uneven amount of caregiving on your part? Ideally, caring for other fully capable people is a two-way street, a mutual sharing of support and nurturing, a collaboration between you and them. While it's completely appropriate to invest a lot of energy in caring for a small child, to largely take over addressing the needs of fully capable people is something else entirely. In some cases, accepting an elevated level of caregiving is actually a way to calm one's own anxiety through exercising control over part of their world. (This control, or course, is just an illusion.) We all like feeling needed, of course, but problems emerge when we are so absorbed in the needs of others that we forget our own. Many of these emerging problems can be food and eating-related.

Worksheet

In your notebook or downloaded "Taking-Care-of-Everyone-but-Me" workbook document, keep track of all the time you spend focused on doing things for other people for at least a week. You needn't log it exactly or minute by minute; a general sense is perfectly fine. The point here is to get a sense of the proportion of time you spend taking care of other people. Remember to consider all of the other relationships in your life, personal as well as professional.

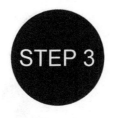

REWORK AND REFRAME

Download the workbook pages for Step Three, or—using the table below as a guide—create the chart in your note book.

	Activity	Time Spent	Satisfaction Level
Example			

In the following week, keep track of the amount of time you spend doing something just for you, including nourishing yourself, moving your body, and allowing quiet time for reading, reflection, or meditation. Also note the quality of the things you do for yourself. How much satisfaction are you deriving from these activities? Is there an obvious lopsidedness in your care efforts that favor other people over your own needs? Additionally, are you taking time for balanced meals and snacks, or grabbing something quick and convenient but not very nutritious? Do you find yourself eating when you are not hungry? Keep track of any such details that might seem relevant.

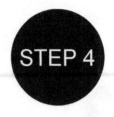

ADJUSTING OLD BEHAVIORS

It's easy to blame cultural pressure for this denial of adequate self-care, but the truth is that much of it is self-imposed. Many women—and some men—want so much to make sure that their world is in order, and the people in their lives are well taken care of, that sometimes the value of their own self-care simply doesn't occur to them. Whether this mindset comes from pressure from our society or an individual's sense of commitment doesn't matter. (It is not unusual for the drive that overcommits caring for others to be rooted in some level of anxiety in the caregiver.) Whether the self-neglect is some sort of self-martyrdom or benign neglectfulness doesn't matter either. What does matter is that this destructive belief assumes that if the caregiver doesn't take care of everybody, all of their loved ones, then they're not a good spouse, parent, child, or friend.

The truth is, of course, that there is no such thing as the perfect spouse, the perfect child, or the perfect parent. Striving for perfection will always come up short. To be good at caring for others requires only empathy and best efforts, not perfection.

It is frequently pointed out that in the event that oxygen masks must be used on airplanes, we must first put the masks on ourselves before assisting children. The reason is simple: to be a responsible caregiver requires that you take care of yourself so that you have the strength—emotional as well as physical—to support those you wish to care for. The takeaway here is that not only should we take care of ourselves because we are worth the effort of self-care, to do otherwise does not serve those we wish to care for in the first place.

Step Four Exercise

This next exercise is very simple: in your notebook or downloaded workbook pages, make a plan to build self-care into your week. As a matter of fact, make self-care your plan on an ongoing basis. Even if you can devote just 15 minutes a day to yourself, it's 15 minutes well spent, as long as these 15 minutes demonstrate your honest, mindful commitment to your own well-being. Here are a few ideas to start you off:

Self-Care Ideas

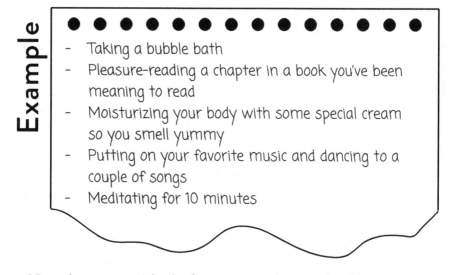

Example

- Taking a bubble bath
- Pleasure-reading a chapter in a book you've been meaning to read
- Moisturizing your body with some special cream so you smell yummy
- Putting on your favorite music and dancing to a couple of songs
- Meditating for 10 minutes

Now it's your turn! Think of ways you might provide self-care. Remember to address each aspect of your daily life: mind/body/spirit.

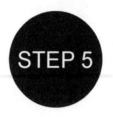

STEP 5

AFFIRM WHO YOU ARE

Some people are so used to short-changing their own needs that to reclaim them feels uncomfortable. Well, being uncomfortable is perfectly okay.

Very often, going through a stage of discomfort is part of expanding into a more complete expression of who you are. With time, embracing this necessary self-care will seem right and good and as comfortable as a cozy blanket.

Obviously, a big part of shifting behavior and expanding comfort levels rests in mindset. We opened this section of appreciating self-care with an affirmation of intent, and now we'll close this chapter with an affirmation of acknowledgement and centering. This final step is an ongoing process to take firm ownership of a new perspective on how to interact with your world.

Take some quiet time to acknowledge this new perspective Then, in your notebook or workbook, write down the following statement, putting your name in the provided blank space.

I am _____. Even as I share my heart with others through my empathy, mindfulness, and care, I remember that I am worthy, and so commit to myself the same empathy, mindfulness, and care ...every day.

Repeat your affirmation to yourself every day in quiet moments, perhaps as you lie in bed in the morning or at the end of your day, or while meditating or exercising. Try to do this every day for at least a month. If you forget, that's fine, just forgive yourself and pick up where you left off. Even if you feel uncomfortable or don't fully believe this statement at first, remember that in order to grow, we must become clear on what we aspire to be.

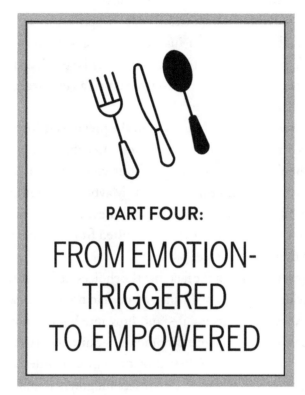

PART FOUR:

FROM EMOTION-TRIGGERED TO EMPOWERED

The Takeaways and General Points all Eaters Need to Hear

The truth is, there are as many kinds of eaters as there are human beings who eat. The Eaters Section (Part Three of this book) was designed around individual categories in order to speak to general types of different eaters. The information in the following section is for everyone, because while personal, food-related issues may be particular to each individual eater and more general eater-group types, a great deal of the ongoing principles of healing are universal.

Ideally, after you worked the steps in the previous section of this book, you are more of an aware and empowered eater than you were when you started the book. You learned more about yourself. You improved your self-talk with a more mindful approach. Maybe you found a way to step past limiting ideas you had about food and eating. You embraced eating intuitively and found your self-talk has shifted from a rule-based "I should really..." to a more empowered "I want to."

It's empowering to own the fact that the choices we face are ours to make. We get to decide if—and how much—we need to nourish ourselves.

Likewise, we get to decide if—and how much—less nourishing food we wish to consume at any given moment. Because the truth is that sometimes a pint of ice cream is our best choice at a time of ordeal. Not the most healthy choice, but so what? If we are less judgmental and more kind to ourselves, we can make room for such choices. After all, we likely make similar choices in other places in our lives.

Haven't you ever bought an extra item of clothing, or a book, or some other impulse item that you don't need but purchased anyway simply because it made you feel good? As long as you don't make such purchases regularly, it likely won't upset your budget. When we let go of "all-or-nothing thinking" and embrace a more flexible approach, making less-than-perfect choices are well within the margin of acceptability. This basic truth is the same with food choices. We are all emotionally triggered from time to time, and for those moments when only less-than-extremely healthy foods will fit the bill...well, let's mindfully enjoy those cookies! And then whenever we are ready, we can mindfully choose to resume eating nourishing food.

No matter the type of eater you might be, preparation is crucial!

There is a cliché that goes, "When you fail to prepare, you prepare to fail." (To be honest, I've always found that expression a bit condescending.) But the saying does contain more than a grain of truth. It reminds us that it is easier to achieve something we wish to achieve if we have a strategy in place. Having a strategy in place includes having all relevant elements ready for use, and makes day-to-day functioning easier. When we are prepared, we are more likely to be ready for whatever shows up. (For example, if I have a working pen by my office phone, I won't need to tell a client sharing critical information to wait while I search for something to write with.)

Being prepared gives us less to have to think about, and helps give us a sense of security that our world is set right. Ensuring we are prepared to the best of our ability is one of the most important forms of self-care and self-support. Personally speaking, feeling unprepared is apt to make me feel at least a little uneasy.

So doesn't it make sense that, in order to maintain a healthy relationship with food, people who are navigating life with eating and food-relationship issues would be well-served by advanced preparedness?

While advance meal-planning is a necessary part of the empowered-eater routine I counsel for many of the eaters in the previous section, making sure you're prepared with food and planned menus is a lifestyle that might as well be universally applied to everyone.

I recommend performing advance meal and snack prep twice a week, and sticking to it. This routine includes creating a menu and then procuring all the ingredients. Set up one major food shop a week, and then a smaller one to fill in additional perishables three or four days later. The more planning that is done in advance, the easier it is to maintain a workable eating strategy. For example, buy or prepare six grilled chicken breasts. Wrap each one individually and place them in the freezer; that way there is always something to defrost to go in a sandwich, dice into a salad, or shred inside a taco. Another food-prep example is to keep cut, pre-washed veggies in a clear container at eye level in the fridge, perhaps with some guacamole or hummus nearby. That way anyone looking for a snack will have something healthy at their fingertips. This method can scale up to fit a family of any size.

Preparation ahead of time is one of the most vital, easiest, and simplest ways to implement and maintain positive eating strategies. Making preparation a habit is a positive predictor for continuing success relative to one's healthy relationship with food.

What We Habitually Tell Ourselves about Ourselves Is Critical

I believe in the power of self-talk. Self-talk helps promote a mindset bias that governs the way we behave. Positive self-talk can guide us to positive self-care, while negative bias can guide us to not-so-great self-care. And the words we use to tell ourselves about ourselves is largely a choice, whether we're aware of that or not. To not actively choose positive self-talk is to open ourselves up to listening to whatever voice is screaming loudest in our heads. More often than not, these voices are the most critical and judgmental, reflecting our anxieties and insecurities. In other words, the voices of negative self-talk.

You may have noticed that affirmations play a significant part in the processes I share in this book. I recommend people renew their positive intentions daily. It is best to do this regularly, whether we are in the mood to recount our great intentions or not. Sometimes we feel very enthusiastic about our intentions while at other times, maybe not so much. In fact, it may be most critical to renew the positive self-talk when we are not feeling particularly positive.

To help keep our self-talk positive and constructive, we would do well to stick to a couple of helpful tools: affirmations and vision boards. I consider these tools emotional-energy investments toward a happier, fuller, more functional life.

Affirmations and Vision Boards

Affirmations and vision boards can be helpful tools. The regular use of affirmations helps to serve as a continuing reminder of, and recommitment to, what one's goals are. When we understand how affirmational thinking works, we can reframe the thoughts we hold about ourselves. We can shift negative, limiting thoughts to more positive, aspirational ones. The use of affirmations is an effective method to keep beneficial intentions sharp. Repeating a positive statement to yourself— silently or out loud—a couple of times a day can yield a tremendous, positive effect. For instance, if someone wants to have greater control over their intake of food they might use an affirmation: "I honor the wisdom of my body and pay attention to the cues that my body alerts me with. I eat when hungry, stop when satisfied, and I am grateful for my food," and say it at least once a day.

A vision board is an artwork version of affirmations, commonly done as cut-out picture collages. Making a vision board or poster of positive words and images to support your intention and conscious thoughts is also a valuable tool toward reminding you what you are manifesting in your life. Making a similar visual reminder as your computer's screen saver can also be a good idea. Anecdotal reports suggest that people who look at a minute of different shots of smiling faces on their computer a few times a day improved their general attitude. What we allow into our consciousness does affect it, for better or worse!

Framing Our Positive Self-Talk

How we frame even our positive self-talk is critically important. One important final note regarding affirmations and vision boards: when creating either affirmations or vision boards, it is critical that the sentiments are phrased in a way that focuses on the positive, not on the negative. Keep things in the present, not in the future. For instance, it is more constructive for the mind to experience the phrase, "I speak calmly and effectively to my kids," than it is to use a phrase like, "I won't yell at my kids." Likewise, "I am eating foods that nourish my body and soul," is recommended over, "I won't eat junk food anymore." As in most cases in life, keeping things positive is always the best approach.

Non-Food Ways to Self-Soothe

As I mentioned earlier in this section, I am not militantly against using food to find comfort, some of the time. I do, however, believe that falling into the habit of using food to self-soothe each and every time we need some comforting is problematic. People who always must have comfort food to be comforted will end up with a relationship with food that is unbalanced and potentially destructive. Having strategies to find comfort in ways other than eating something is crucial.

Earlier we discussed the importance of preparation in sustaining a good relationship with food, and this kind of forethought is also key in having non-food ways to self-soothe close at hand. It is a good idea to have something standing by for those occasions that call for something to do for comfort. You may have thought of some things you might do to soothe yourself that don't involve food; I have put together a list of suggested activities to add to those ideas:

- Exercise/gentle movement (it releases endorphins)
- Writing in your journal
- Engage in heart-felt prayer
- Coloring in a coloring book for grown-ups
- Taking up a hobby such as knitting, needlepoint, or needle-felting
- Nature walks through woods or a beach
- Playing with a loving pet
- Dancing or singing along to upbeat music you like
- Engaging your mind: jigsaw, crossword, word-search, sudoku puzzles, etc.
- Shoot baskets or practice putting golf balls
- Practicing meditation to soothing music
- Taking a relaxing bath, surrounded by candles and soft music
- Making a list of things you're grateful for
- Assembling a gratitude board by making a collage of things in your life you're grateful for
- Saying your affirmations
- Making and then admiring your vision boards

- Putting on nice-smelling cream
- Reaching out and talking to a person you trust
- Reconnecting with an old friend who makes your heart smile when you think about them
- Listening to an interesting subject on podcasts (one that doesn't raise your anxiety level)
- Reading for pleasure
- Treating yourself to a foot massage or use an electric massaging foot-bath
- Enjoying 20 minutes of yoga exercises, whether on a chair or on a mat (Free instructional videos are available for download or streaming from the Integrating Nutrition website, integratingnutrition.com.)
- Lighting a scented candle: citrus, lavender, and jasmine seem to elevate moods
- Closing your eyes and visualizing things that currently make you happy or you aspire to
- Closing your eyes and listening to pre-recorded guided imagery that you pre-recorded or downloaded from this book's website

And finally...hooray!

My goal in writing this book was to include as much useful information and guidance as possible to help my readers heal their relationship with food. While it is up to you, of course, to do the (sometimes very challenging) real work, I hope you found this book clearly written and the guidance helpful and easy to follow.

I'd like to offer you my heartfelt congratulations. You took charge of your relationship with eating and with food; by facing these issues, you demonstrated a renewed commitment to yourself. Please remember that it is enough for you to do your best, and sometimes doing your best is less than perfect. We all need to give ourselves a break when we drop the ball now and then, so by all means...let us *not* get hung up on perfection.

~Lisa Ellis

For printable versions of the tools and solutions presented in this book, as well as helpful additional materials, visit www.whydidijusteat-that.com and click on the RESOURCES tab.

ABOUT THE AUTHOR

Lisa D. Ellis, MS, RDN, CDN, LCSW, CEDS-C (she/her) is a Registered Dietitian, Certified Eating Disorders Specialist and IAEDP Approved Consultant, and therapist. Areas of expertise include eating disorders and emotion-triggered eating. She received a B.S. in nutrition and psychology from Simmons University, an M.S. in clinical nutrition from New York Medical College, and an MSW from Fordham University. Her warm and 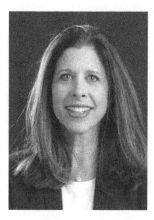 friendly approach and her deep understanding of the emotional and psychological aspects of eating disorders have made her a trusted voice in the field. As the founder of Integrating Nutrition in Manhattan and Westchester County, NY, Lisa helps people heal their relationships with food by shifting their nutritional approach from diet-based pressure and shame...to empowerment.

NOTES

The Pendulum Eater

1   Hall, K. D., & Kahan, S. (2018). Maintenance of lost weight and long-term management of obesity. The Medical Clinics of North America, 102(1), 183. https://doi.org/10.1016/j.mcna.2017.08.012

2   Doran, George (1981) There's a S.M.A.R.T. way to write management goals and objectives. Management Review. 11/81 35–36. https://community.mis.temple.edu/mis0855002fall2015/files/2015/10/S.M.A.R.T-Way-Management-Review.pdf

The Sleep-Deprived Snacker

3   Soltanieh, S., Solgi, S., Ansari, M., Santos, H. O., & Abbasi, B. (2021). Effect of sleep duration on dietary intake, desire to eat, measures of food intake and metabolic hormones: A systematic review of clinical trials. Clinical Nutrition ESPEN, 45, 55-65. https://doi.org/10.1016/j.clnesp.2021.07.029

4   Csipo, T., Lipecz, A., Owens, C., Mukli, P., Perry, J. W., Tarantini, S., Balasubramanian, P., Yabluchanska, V., Sorond, F. A., Kellawan, J. M., Purebl, G., Sonntag, W. E., Csiszar, A., Ungvari, Z., & Yabluchanskiy, A. (2021). Sleep deprivation impairs cognitive performance, alters task-associated cerebral blood flow and decreases cortical neurovascular coupling-related hemodynamic responses. Scientific Reports, 11(1), 1-13. https://doi.org/10.1038/s41598-021-00188-8

A free ebook edition is available with the purchase of this book.

To claim your free ebook edition:

1. Visit MorganJamesBOGO.com
2. Sign your name CLEARLY in the space
3. Complete the form and submit a photo of the entire copyright page
4. You or your friend can download the ebook to your preferred device

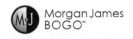

Morgan James
BOGO™

A **FREE** ebook edition is available for you or a friend with the purchase of this print book.

CLEARLY SIGN YOUR NAME ABOVE

Instructions to claim your free ebook edition:
1. Visit MorganJamesBOGO.com
2. Sign your name CLEARLY in the space above
3. Complete the form and submit a photo of this entire page
4. You or your friend can download the ebook to your preferred device

Print & Digital Together Forever.

Snap a photo

Free ebook

Read anywhere

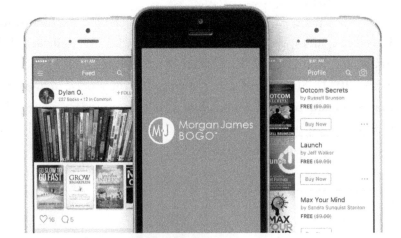